M.R. Ahuja received his Ph.D. in genetics from the University of California, Berkeley, USA. While working for his doctorate and subsequently too, Dr. Ahuja has been interested in the genetic mechansims that control the differentiation of cells into normal or cancerous types. In particular, his research has centred on the role of genetic components and environmental factors in the origin of cancer. He has worked for a number of years at the Institute of Cancer Research, Philadelphia, USA. Later, Dr. Ahuja held various posts such as professor of genetics at the Pant University of Agriculture and Technology, Pantnagar, India and visiting professor at the Institute of Genetics, University of Giessen, Germany. Currently he is the head of Molecular Genetics and Genetics Engineering at the Institute of Forest Genetics, Grosshansdorf, Germany.

CANCER
Causes and Prevention

Dr. M.R. Ahuja

UBSPD

UBS Publishers' Distributors Ltd.

New Delhi • Mumbai • Bangalore • Chennai
Calcutta • Patna • Kanpur • London

UBS Publishers' Distributors Ltd.

5 Ansari Road, New Delhi-110 002
Phones : 3273601, 3266646 ☆ *Cable* : ALLBOOKS ☆
Fax : (91) 11-327-6593
E-mail: ubspd.del@smy.sprintrpg.ems.vsnl.net.in
Apeejay Chambers, 5 Wallace Street, Mumbai-400 001
Phones : 2046971, 2047700 ☆ *Cable* : UBSIPUB ☆
Fax : 2040827
10 First Main Road, Gandhi Nagar, Bangalore-560 009
Phones : 2263901, 2263902, 2253903 ☆ *Cable* : ALLBOOKS ☆
Fax : 2263904
6, Sivaganga Road, Nungambakkam, Chennai-600 034
Phone : 8276355 ☆ *Cable* : UBSIPUB ☆ *Fax* : 8270189
8/1-B, Chowringhee Lane, Calcutta-700 016
Phones : 2441821, 2442910, 2449473 ☆ *Cable* : UBSIPUBS ☆
Fax : 2450027
5 A, Rajendra Nagar, Patna-800 016
Phones : 652856, 653973, 656170 ☆ *Cable* : UBSPUB ☆
Fax : 656169
80, Noronha Road, Cantonment, Kanpur-208 004
Phones : 369124, 362665, 357488 ☆ *Fax* : 315122

First Published 1997

Cover illustration : Ila Ahuja
Cover design : UBS Art Studio

Designed & Typeset at UBSPD in 11 pt Souvenir
Printed at Replika Press Pvt. Ltd., Delhi-110 033 (India

To
The memory of Dr. Jack Schultz,
my mentor

Preface

This book has been written for a broad spectrum of society, including the educated public and health professionals interested in the cancer problem. Those students seeking a career in cancer research will also find the book informative. I have attempted to keep the text as simple as possible and have avoided unnecessary details and lapses into technicalities. But in a book on such a topic as cancer, it is sometimes difficult to avoid complex terminology.

I have provided a broad coverage of the cancer problem, including the nature of the disease, the probable causes, the importance of genetic and environmental factors in the origin of cancer, the detection, the treatment, the prevention, the genetic counselling for the cancer probands and individuals at a high risk of hereditary cancers, experimental systems and new perspectives in cancer research, and finally the origin and the evolution of cancer genes. In particular, this book deals with (1) the genetic nature of cancer, (2) the prevalence of potentially carcinogenic substances in the human environment and their interaction with the host's genome, (3) the essential biological and biochemical differences between a cancer cell and its normal counterpart in terms of phenotype and the degree of differentiation, and (4) how this basic knowledge may lead us to develop approaches towards prevention and eventual control of cancer.

In this book it is not my intention to draw the reader's attention either to the suffering and misery of human cancer or to the costs involved in its treatment. Also, for that matter, I do not propose to dwell on the pathogenesis of the disease. Instead, I have included chapters on the role of genetics and environmental factors, customs, habits and diet in human cancer, and strategies to prevent this disease. In doing so, I have not neglected to retain the current thinking in contemporary biology relevant to the cancer problem, since it will be through acquiring a better knowledge of normal cellular processes involved in cell reproduction and cell differentiation that we will come closer to an understanding of the causes and origin of cancer.

The genesis of this book can be traced to the Institute of Genetics, University of Giessen, Germany, where I spent two years as a visiting professor and later several years as a geneticist, almost two decades ago. Ever since, I have been working on this project, trying to keep up with the recent developments in cancer research and cell differentiation. In between the AIDS (acquired immunodeficiency syndrome) virus was discovered and the worldwide dangers of this scourge and associated cancers have assumed alarming proportions. The concepts and ideas on tumour genes, regulatory genes, the oncogenes, anti-oncogenes, and the tumour suppressor genes, also added new dimensions to cancer research. All these features as well as new discoveries in genetic engineering made the task of completing this book somewhat difficult but more challenging.

This book is born out of my personal experience extending over several decades in cancer genetics starting as a graduate student in the Department of Genetics, University of California, Berkeley, USA, continuing at the Institute of Cancer Research, Fox Chase, Philadelphia, USA, and later at the Institute of Genetics, University of Giessen, Germany. My discussions with a number of colleagues and students provided a greater impetus for the continuation of this project. In particular, I would like to thank Drs. Fritz Anders (Giessen), William J. Libby (Berkeley), Everett R. Dempster (Berkeley), Grant Doering (Philadelphia), Ernst Caspari (Rochester), and Manfred Schwab (Giessen) for stimulating discussions in cancer research. Of course, I am solely responsible for the contents of this book.

I wrote parts of the book in Giessen, continued to do so in Mombasa, Kenya, later in Grosshansdorf, Germany, and finally completed the text in Philadelphia. During this writing spree, my family and I had a very pleasant stay in Kenya. I am grateful to Prem and Amala Prinja for according us splendid hospitality in their beautifully located mansion on the Nyali beach in Mombasa. Finally, I am thankful to my daughter Hemna for the graphics, and indebted to my wife Ila for suggesting a number of improvements in the text and in the artworks, and for being a constant source of inspiration throughout the preparation of this book.

Dr. M. R. Ahuja

Contents

Preface *vii*

1. Introduction **1**

2. A Normal Cell and a Cancer Cell **7**
Structure of a Normal Cell 8
Differences between Normal and Cancer Cells 12
Benign and Malignant Tumour Cells 13
Cell Type and Cancer 14

3. The Structure and Expression of Genes **16**
Genes and Traits 16
Composition of a Gene 17
Genes in Cell Division 18
Genes in Action 20
Mutation 26

4. The Cell Cycle and Cancer **28**
The Four Periods of the Cell Cycle 28
Variable and Constant Components of the Cell Cycle 30
The Cell Division 31
G1 Period and Cell Proliferation 34

Normal Cells Behave Like Cancer Cells during Regeneration 36
Continuous and Uncontrolled Cell Reproduction in Cancer Cells 37

5. Cell Differentiation and Cancer **39**
Growth and Differentiation in the Human Embryo and an Adult 40
Differentiation: A Heritable and Well-Coordinated Process 41
Clonal Origin of Cancer 42

6. Genes and Human Cancer **47**
Genetic and Environmental Factors 47
Genetic Predisposition to Cancer 53
Genetic Defects and the Time Course of Hereditary Cancer 60
Chromosome Abnormalities and Cancer 61
Chromosome Aberrations May Cause Impairment of Suppressor Genes 65

7. Environmental Factors and Cancer (I) **67**
Occupations, Customs and Habits 67
Occupational Cancers 69
Cancers Associated with Customs and Habits 71

8. Environmental Factors and Cancer (II) **73**
Tobacco, Diet, and Other Potentially Carcinogenic Substances 73
Tobacco 74
Diet 76
Potentially Carcinogenic Substances for Humans 82

9. Environmental Factors and Cancer (III) **88**
Chemical Carcinogens 88
Conversion of Chemical Carcinogens into an Active Form 89
Screening of Chemicals for Carcinogenicity 91
Chemical Carcinogenesis: Initiation and Promotion 92
Mechanisms of Chemical Carcinogenesis 94

10. Environmental Factors and Cancer (IV) **95**
Radiation 95
Atomic Bombs and Cancer 96
Nuclear Accidents and Cancer 98
Ultraviolet Radiation and Radioactive Substances 99
Mammography 100
Microwave Radiation 100
The Effect of Radiation on Cells 101
Forms of Radiation and Cancer 103

11. Viruses, Oncogenes and Cancer **105**
Oncogenic and Non-Oncogenic Viruses 105
Structure and Reproduction of Viruses 106
The Host Range of Viruses 108
DNA Tumour Viruses 109
RNA Tumour Viruses 112
AIDS 120
Transformation of Cells by Viruses 122

12. Aging and Cancer **125**
What Is Aging? 125
Association between Aging and Cancer 128

13. The Origin of Cancer **129**
The Mutation Concept 130
The Epigenetic Concept 132
The Viral Concept 132
A Unified Genetic Concept of Cancer 133

14. Experimental Systems in Cancer Research **139**
The Crown Gall System 140
The Genetic Tumour System in Tobacco 141
The Platyfish-Swordtail System 144
The Mouse System 149
The Human System 153
Normal Cells and Cancer Cells *in vitro* 154

15. Detection of Cancer **158**
Cancer Warning Signals 159
Biochemical Markers for Early Detection of Cancer 159

Markers in Blood 160
Markers in Urine 162

16. Strategies for the Control of Human Cancer 164
Treatment of Cancer 165
Biological Therapy (Immunotherapy) 171

17. Prevention of Cancer 174
Tobacco Smoking 176
Sunlight (Ultraviolet Rays) 177
Diet 177
Ionizing Radiation 179
Alcohol, Drugs, and Promiscuity 179
Lifestyle and Cancer Prevention 181

18. Genetic Counselling for Hereditary Cancers 183
Cancer of the Colon 184
Xeroderma Pigmentosum 185
Prospects for Genetic Counselling 186

19. New Perspectives in Cancer Research 188
Fusion of Malignant and Normal Cells 189
Jumping Genes and Cancer 190
Cell Death and Immortality 191
Cell Cycle Genes in Cancer 194
Regulatory Genes and Suppressor Genes 195
Genome Structure and Mapping 197
Genetic Engineering and Cancer 199

20. Origin and Evolution of Cancer Genes 201
The Replicator 201
Ontogeny of Cancer Genes 203

Epilogue *207*
Select Bibliography *211*
Index *221*

1

Introduction

Cancer is a disease of cells – living cells – in the multicellular organisms, and as long as there are living cells that are capable of division, there exists the possibility that they might become cancerous. What a commentary on life! But that seems to be the *Tao* of cells. In this context, cancer is a very old disease, and may have had its origins when the multicellular organisms evolved, much before the dinosaurs or even their evolutionary ancestors traversed our planet. Our knowledge on cancer goes back to the dawn of civilization. Perhaps the earliest records of the disease may be traced to the ancient Egyptian, Indian and Greek writings, in which some rational methods of treatment/control, then available, were described. For example, the ancient Egyptians practised a 'fire drill' (hyperthermia), which involved insertion of a heated stick into the tumours to treat them.

The modern era of pathology began following the invention of the microscope. This instrument opened man's eyes to a vast new world of living forms, including cells, previously not available to observation and study. Microbes were discovered and relationships between disease-causing microbes and abnormalities of cells of the body were recognized. It was also discovered, in the sphere of cancer, that the affected tissues were also composed of living cells and these cancer cells were originally derived from normal cells of the body.

The living organisms are composed of cells which are programmed to fulfil certain functions. The normal cell reproduction and multiplication are controlled and restrained. But sometimes certain factor(s) initiate(s) a genetic change which disrupts the normal cell function and forces it to behave abnormally. It appears as though the controls and restraints for normal growth and differentiation have vanished. The end result is that the new abnormal or cancer cell possesses certain invasive characteristics. The striking difference is that cancer cells, unlike their normal counterparts, fail to be governed by normal controls and undergo unrestrained cell reproduction. In short, cancer cells behave in a chaotic manner. The cells' information centre appears to be relaying garbled messages which disorient them and affect their function. They start multiplying in a haphazard and unrestrained manner. The cancer cells do not obey any restrictions or boundaries and aggressively invade their progenitor's normal cells and the surrounding tissues and destroy them. What could have gone wrong? What caused the normal cells to become self-destructive? This is a mystery that still remains to be resolved.

Cancer occurs in different forms in different tissues, and is often said to include a large variety of diseases. For example, cancer of the white blood cells (leukaemia) has no resemblance to cancer of the stomach, lung, or brain. Although, superficially, there seems to be little resemblance between cancers of different tissues of organs, most cancers share some common biological properties, such as unrestrained cell reproduction, lack of cell maturation, invasive behaviour, and a loss of normal cellular function. Cancer strikes, with equally devastating force, all forms of higher organisms – plants, fishes, dogs, cows, and humans, to mention a few. All cancer cells are derived from normal cells, and these may include skin, lung, intestine, brain, bone, spleen or blood cells. Once the normal cells have been transformed into cancerous cells, they multiply at a relatively fast rate and lose all restraints and controls vital to coordinated growth and differentiation of normal cells. In the advanced stages, the cancer cells invade and destroy the surrounding normal tissues, often accompanied by metastasis (migration) via the blood stream and lymph channels to other parts of the body.

There are a number of warning signals or symptoms which might indicate the onset of cancer. However, these may also be caused by other medical problems. Therefore, detection of cancer in the early stages is often problematic. In most other human ailments there are certain specific symptoms which identify the microbe-host relationship to a fair degree and thus help in prescribing a cure. For instance, when staphylococcus bacteria attack the skin cells, there is a detectable inflammation accompanied by pain. In case of a malarial attack, the malarial parasite causes high fever with general soreness of the body. There are ups and downs in body temperature, and the temperature peaks coincide with certain reproductive phases of the malarial parasite in the blood stream. In contrast to the aforementioned general situations, cancer in itself is not painful in the initial stages and it may exist for a long time without causing the least trouble or apprehension. It is precisely this insidious nature of the disease that makes it dangerous; a feature that delays its early diagnosis and hence the timely institution of appropriate treatment. It appears that in most cancers, there is a prolonged 'latent period' which may elapse between the initial cause and the appearance of the cancer or tumour. This latent period may range anywhere from 5 to 15 years in human beings.

The causes of cancer have not been completely understood at the present time. However, several lines of experimental evidence suggest a multifactor involvement. A number of diverse environmental factors, such as X-rays, ultraviolet rays, chemicals, and viruses, seem to be involved in the aetiology of cancer. Although the precise mechanisms of transformation of a normal cell to a cancer cell are not yet well understood, it seems highly plausible that these diverse environmental factors, singly or in combination, may, in a great majority of cases, directly or indirectly, affect the genetic components of the cell to cause a certain genetic change which has relevance to the origin of cancer. Since the daughter cells exhibit properties similar to the progenitor cancer cell, cancer is generally believed to be a genetic disease involving lesions at the biochemical and molecular levels.

This book critically examines the role of both the environmental factors and the genetic factors in the development of cancer, in particular, human cancer. It has been variously estimated that 75 per cent to 90 per cent of human cancers are due to environmental carcinogens and, in principle, preventable. Since cancer is a genetic condition, that is, cancer cells carry defective genes, it becomes important to identify environmental factors that cause the cancer-related genetic changes in the normal cells. For instance, there is a strong relationship between cigarette smoking and lung cancer. Therefore, lung cancer may be largely prevented in susceptible individuals by giving up smoking. Diet has been implicated in the cancer of the stomach and the large intestine. Therefore, identification of specific ingredients in diet may lead to a better understanding about the diet-cancer relationship.

There are several human cancers whose predispositions are controlled in inheritance by one or two genes. But even in these cases, environmental factors do play a role, however small, in the expression and development of cancer. For example, patients with Xeroderma pigmentosum, a recessive genetic defect, are at a high risk of developing skin cancer when exposed to sunlight. Preventive measures involve either keeping away from sunlight or wearing appropriate clothing for protection against ultraviolet rays. In some other cancers whose predisposition is controlled by relatively few genes, we have to learn more about the gene action and microenvironmental factors (intrinsic and extrinsic) involved in these cancers before attempting to consider control measures.

It should be mentioned though that genetic aberrations are common in normal cells. But all genetic changes do not lead to the onset of cancer. In fact, a large number of aberrations are repaired by the living cells, and it is a very small proportion of these genetic changes that lead to genetic diseases, including cancer. But cancer distinguishes itself from other genetic diseases, such as sickle cell anaemia or Huntington's chorea, by specific genetic alterations which initiate unrestrained cell divisions, accompanied by invasive behaviour. The aggressive cancer cells push their way through the normal ancestral cells and unabatedly destroy them. Destruction of cells by foreign intruders, such as microbes, is not uncommon. But cells killing their own kind is something quite different. Creation and destruction are the two opposing forces whose balance is necessary for the preservation of life. In cancer, the balance seems to be tipped in favour of destruction.

Although early detection of the disease remains a challenging problem in cancer research, the current search for biochemical markers in blood and urine is a step in the right direction. Indexing of all the proteins in the human body (some 30,000 to 50,000), when completed, may make it possible some day to detect abnormal activities of certain proteins that may be associated with the early development of specific human cancers.

More recently, the 'DNA fingerprinting' (polymorphic DNA markers that differ between individuals) technique has been developed for analysis of the human genome by employing a polymerase chain reaction (PCR). DNA fingerprints can serve as unique genetic markers for locating defective genes in inherited diseases, including hereditary cancers. When the DNA of an individual is chopped with one or more restriction enzymes (enzymes that cut the DNA chain at specific sites), a set of DNA fragments of various sizes are produced. This restriction fragment length polymorphism (RFLP) may be exploited to establish whether or not a particular locus is associated with a disease, simply by comparing DNA restriction fragment data of healthy and afflicted individuals from a number of different but affected families. By employing this approach, it has been possible to determine the general location of the gene involved in Huntington's chorea on a specific chromosome in the human genome. Similarly, sites of other genes on human chromosomes, involved in a number of inherited diseases, have been determined. In this direction, the human genome project currently underway will provide a complete repository of our normal and defective genes.

When cancer is detected in the early stages, the cure rates will also be reasonably high. The current methods of treatment are not very effective for most varieties of human cancer because, in a majority of cases, the cancers, when discovered, are already in advanced stages of development and have already undergone metastasis, that is, the cancer has already spread from one part or organ to another part of the body.

One of the major objectives of cancer research is to find out what causes the transformation of a normal cell into a cancer cell. The key to the secret of this conversion from the normal state to the cancerous state is believed to lie within each normal cell. Therefore, research in cell biology, particularly molecular biology, pertaining to cell reproduction and cell differentiation, may lead us some day to understand cancer *in toto* and conquer it.

2

A Normal Cell and a Cancer Cell

The cell is the basic unit of the tissues and the organs that make up the bodies of the multicellular organisms. The morphology of cells varies in different tissues, depending upon the type of specialized function a cell might perform in a certain tissue. However, all living cells consist of a spherical body, called the nucleus, which is usually located centrally, surrounded by a viscous fluid called the cytoplasm. The outermost envelope of the cytoplasm is the plasma membrane. The plasma membrane acts as a selective sieve, and allows only a controlled movement of molecules across this barrier, from one cell to another or from the surrounding medium into the cell. Each cell is like a minifactory and has a blueprint for producing material for its own use: for example, reproduction, or in a specialized case, making growth hormones or digestive enzymes that are transported outside the cell in the blood stream or the stomach. Thus, the body is composed of different types of cells producing different products essential for the normal structure and function of the organs in a body.

STRUCTURE OF A NORMAL CELL

Since the very existence of all living organisms is dependent on cells, it is important to understand their structure and function. Most cells are too small to be seen with the naked eye, and hence there is a necessity to magnify them in order to examine their structure. The unaided human eye has a resolving power of about 0.1 millimetre or 100 μ (1 millimetre = 1000 μ). In the light microscope one can see objects down to about 0.5 μ, while the resolving limit of the electron microscope is about 0.001 μ. In other words, if the human eye has a resolving power of 1, then that of the light microscope is 500, and that of an electron microscope approaches 100,000. The electron microscope has thus opened up a whole new domain to the cytologists by allowing them to examine a number of subcellular structures and organelles. The structure of a typical animal cell is shown in Fig. 2.1.

Cytoplasm

There are several organelles in the cytoplasm which must carry out the 'housekeeping' job of the cell by performing useful functions to keep the cell alive. One of the essential requirements is the energy to support the activities of the cell. This energy is generated by small vesicles called mitochondria present in the cytoplasm. Each cell contains a large number of mitochondria, which break down sugars and other energy-rich molecules to release energy. Another cellular task is the production of proteins, which is performed by extremely small particles called ribosomes, and there are several thousands of these in a cell. The ribosomes may be attached to a system of cytoplasmic membranes called endoplasmic reticulum, or they may be free-floating in the cytoplasmic fluid. This fluid contains a large number of different kinds of molecules that seem to be involved in important cellular functions. In particular, many of these

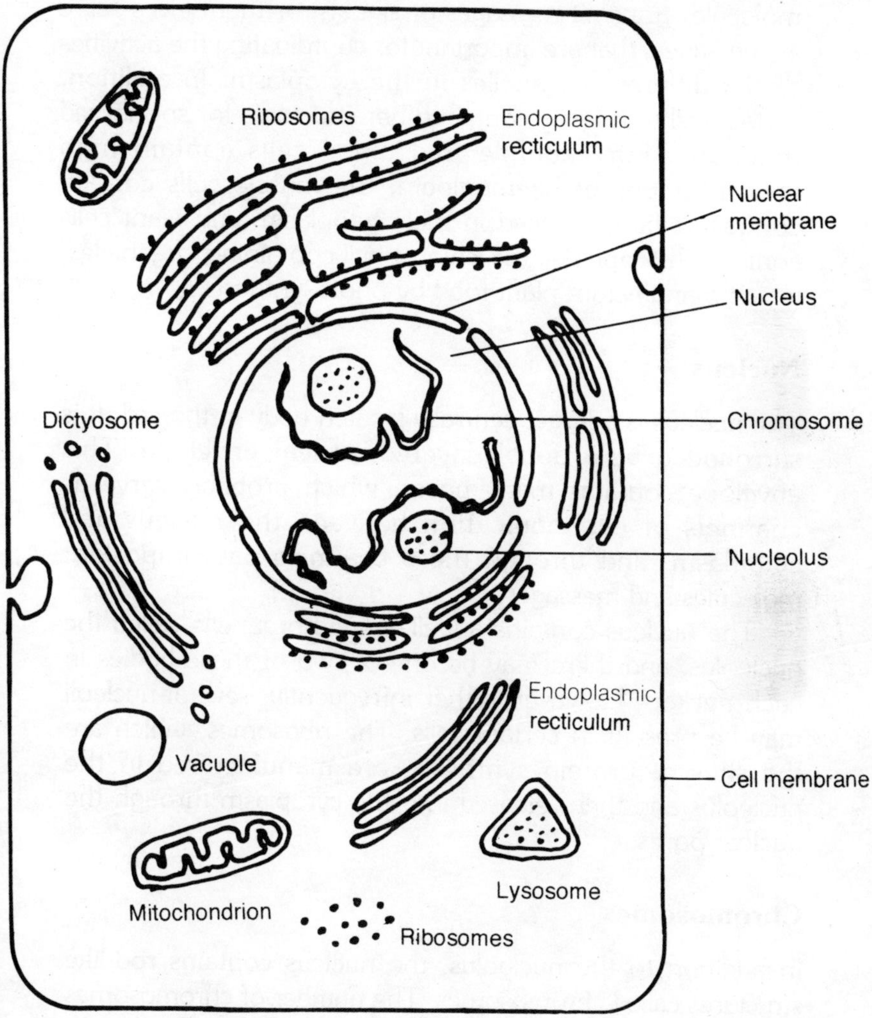

Fig. 2.1 **Structure of an animal cell. In the centre of the cell is a circular body called the nucleus, which controls the cell's activities. Messages are passed on from the nucleus through the pores in the nuclear membrane into the cytoplasm for coordination of various cellular activities, including the synthesis of proteins and enzymes required for life functions.**

molecules transmit messages or signals, or themselves serve as messages, that are important for coordinating the activities of the different organelles in the cytoplasm. In addition, certain cell types may contain other structures for specialized functions. For example: red blood cells contain high concentrations of haemoglobin; the muscle cells contain contractile fibres packed in their cytoplasm; and plant cells contain chloroplasts, the chlorophyll-containing organelles, which manufacture plant food by photosynthesis.

Nucleus

The nucleus is a large, centrally located body in the cell. It is surrounded by a double-layered nuclear envelope. This envelope contains many pores, which probably serve as channels of communication between the nucleus and cytoplasm, and through these channels pass important molecules and messages.

The nucleus contains a well-defined organelle called the nucleolus, and there may be one or two of these bodies in each nucleus. However, rather infrequently, several nucleoli may be present in certain cells. The ribosomes, which are the sites of protein synthesis, are manufactured in the nucleolus and then released into the cytoplasm through the nuclear pores.

Chromosomes

In addition to the nucleolus, the nucleus contains rod-like structures called chromosomes. The number of chromosomes per nucleus is, as a rule, characteristic for the cells of each particular species. For example, the normal chromosome number in humans is 46 (Fig. 2.2), in the gorilla and the chimpanzee 48, in the rhesus monkey 42, in the rabbit 44, in the mouse 40, and in the hamster 22. The chromosomes are present in pairs, but with the exception of XY sex chromosomes, the members of a pair of chromosomes cannot be normally distinguished under the light microscope. Thus, human beings have 23 pairs of chromosomes, and the gorilla and the chimpanzee have 24 pairs. Generally, however, each pair of chromosomes can be distinguished from each other in man. Based on the length and morphology (position of the centromere or the constriction), the 46 human chromosomes are divided into

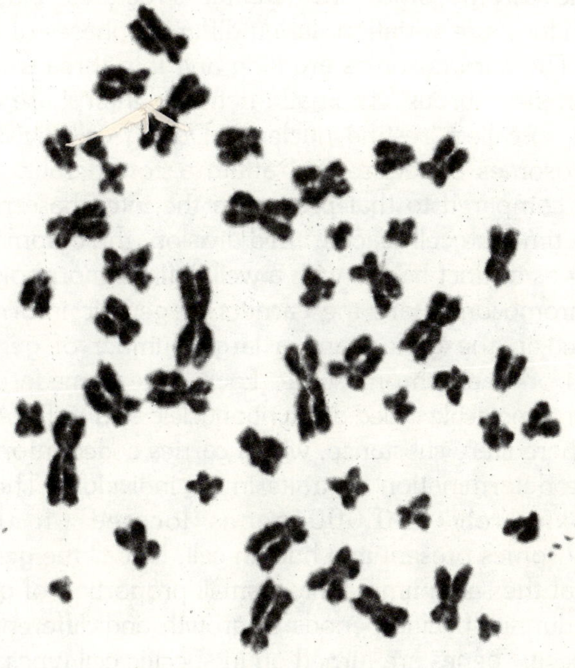

Fig. 2.2 **A photograph showing 46 human chromosomes. The chromosome pairs are distinguishable on the basis of the length and position of the centromere (constriction). The chromosomes are the carriers of the genetic information coded in the genes for different traits; for example, eye colour, height, facial characters, and blood group. Genes that prevent cancer (suppressor genes) and those involved in cancer (oncogenes) are also located on the chromosomes.**

seven groups designated from A to G: A group being the longest and G the shortest, and the remaining in between. The distribution of chromosomes in these seven groups is as follows: A group (three pairs), B group (two pairs), C group (seven pairs) and an X chromosome in male, or eight pairs including XX chromosomes in the female, D group (three pairs), E group (three pairs), F group (two pairs), and G group (two pairs and the Y chromosome).

The chromosomes are dynamic structures undergoing tremendous size variation during different phases of the cell cycle. The chromosomes are long and thin threads forming the complex fibrous 'chromatin network' interphase nucleus or the so-called 'resting nucleus'. During cell division the chromosomes condense and attain a considerably shorter length compared to that present in the interphase nucleus. By the time the cell reaches mid-division, the chromosomes appear as distinct bodies with a well-defined morphology.

Chromosomes are the carriers of genetic information, encoded in the genes, and a large number of genes are located on each chromosome. Each gene is made up of a very long molecule called deoxyribonucleic acid or DNA. DNA is the hereditary substance, which carries coded information for the determination of traits in an individual. There are approximately 100,000 genes located on the 46 chromosomes present in a human cell. Not all the genes are active at the same time. Only a small proportion of genes is active during specific periods of growth and differentiation, and specific genes are turned on in specific cell types.

DIFFERENCES BETWEEN NORMAL AND CANCER CELLS

Numerous studies have been conducted to find out differences in the structure of normal *vs*. cancer cells. In earlier studies, where normal mature cells were used as controls, it appeared as though there might be differences in the cell morphology, the nuclear-cytoplasmic ratio, and the structure of subcellular organelles, such as endoplasmic reticulum and mitochondria. However, these differences turned out to be superficial when comparisons were made between cancer cells and the normal growing counterpart cells. It has become increasingly clear that there are no major *structural* differences between cancer cells and their normal counterpart growing cell types. On the other hand, a cancer cell differs from a normal cell in *function* and *behaviour*. By and large, the cancer cells do not perform any useful function for an individual, as opposed to the normal cells that are involved in the manufacture of proteins and enzymes for keeping us alive. Instead, the cancer cells are invasive in their behaviour and destroy surrounding normal cells and tissues, and migrate (metastasize) via the blood stream to distant parts of the body and set up new cancer cell colonies. This invasive and naked aggression of the cancer cells is a single most devastating force, which not only destroys useful cells of the body, but, in the final stages, becomes uncontrollable by any iatrogenic weaponry available in human hands. The death of an individual occurs when one or more vital tissues/organs in the body have been destroyed by the cancer cells.

BENIGN AND MALIGNANT TUMOUR CELLS

It appears that nearly every living cell, capable of division, in the body has the potential of being transformed into a cancer cell. What a bleak and depressing picture, especially when one considers the fact that a human body consists of approximately 100 plus cell types. In simple terms, this would mean that about 100 distinct varieties of cancer could occur. But fortunately most of these cancers are rare. The three organs mainly afflicted by cancer are the lung, the large intestine and the breast. It is estimated that they account for roughly half the cancer deaths. Therefore, it is imperative to focus research on the understanding of the cellular structure and function. Why do normal cells lose their direction, multiply haphazardly and form tumours which have only one goal and that is destruction of normal cells leading to the death of the organism? Why do normal living cells have genes for self-destruction? Is it that creation and destruction are two sides of the same coin, and that both must exist in complete harmony and balance? Is this the Cosmic Law of the Universe? Any disturbance in this equilibrium could result in chaos and disorientation of cells and in eventual death. One of those chaotic manifestations of normal cells leading to irreparable damage may be the formation of tumours.

Tumours can originate in any part of the body. There are two broad categories of tumours: (a) those that remain localized and do not invade the surrounding normal tissues are called *benign* tumours and (b) those that are invasive and spread from their site of origin to other parts of the body through the lymphatic system and blood stream are called *malignant* tumours or cancers. When a normal cell is transformed into a cancer cell, there occur profound heritable changes which allow the cancer cell to largely determine its own activities, such as continuous cell division, aberrant cell differentiation, and invasive behaviour, against which there is no adequate control mechanism in the host. Thus, a cancer cell is a genetically altered cell, as compared to the normal cells from which it is derived, and when the cancer cell divides, it transmits its new attributes to its daughter cells.

CELL TYPE AND CANCER

Based on the cell type/tissue of their origin, most of the human cancers may be classified into three major groups: namely, carcinomas, sarcomas, and a heterogeneous group, including leukaemias. Carcinoma is a type of cancer that originates in the covering tissue (epithelial cells); for example, skin, intestine, respiratory tract, and also in the lining of various glands, such as breast, thyroid, or pancreas.

Sarcomas develop in the cells of the connective tissues, such as bone, cartilage, fatty tissue, and fibrous tissues. The heterogeneous group includes leukaemias, lymphomas, and lymphosarcomas. Leukaemia is a cancer resulting from uncontrolled proliferation of white blood cells (leucocytes), and lymphomas include cancers of the immune system (lymphocytes). Carcinomas and sarcomas are solid tumours, while leukaemias, which represent excess circulating cancer cells, do not form solid tumours. Of the three groups of cancers, carcinomas seem to be the most prevalent type representing more than 90 per cent of human cancers. Sarcomas and leukaemias are far less prevalent and constitute less than 10 per cent of the human cancers. The preponderance of carcinomas may be due to the fact that the covering tissues come in direct contact with environmental factors that may initiate cancer.

And finally, cancers may also be classified according to an organ, site and cell type. For example: retinoblastoma, which originates in the retinal cells, is a highly malignant tumour of the eye; Xeroderma pigmentosum, in which the skin is highly sensitive to sunlight and develops multiple tumours; and melanoma, a cancer arising from the pigment cells of the deep layers of the skin.

In all types of cancer, the ultimate target of the environmental carcinogens seems to be the cell's genetic material; the environmental agents cause a certain genetic change. This change may involve defective genes and/or chromosomal abnormalities. The genetic factors (genes) and cancer will be discussed in more detail in Chapter 6.

3

The Structure and Expression of Genes

GENES AND TRAITS

Chromosomes are the vehicles that carry hereditary information from one generation to the next. Genetic information is encoded in the genes and a large number of them are located in a linear order on each chromosome. The normal human complement of 46 chromosomes carries hundreds of thousands of genes. There may be more than 100,000 genes in the human genome. Genes are the determinants of various traits in our body: for example, eye colour, colour vision, blood clotting, the blood groups (A, B, or O), the Rhesus factor (Rh), height, size and shape of our eyes, nose, lips, arms, torso and legs. Genes also determine an individual's sensitivity to the herpes virus and the polio virus, susceptibility to cancer, and to a host of other human diseases. In other words, besides determining different cellular functions and body attributes, some genes also provide resistance protection against cancer and other diseases. In addition, genes are directly involved in supplying instructions for the manufacture of life-supporting products, the proteins and enzymes. Another function of the genes is to control the amount of proteins to be manufactured at a given time in an organ. They also determine whether or not a certain protein is to be produced at all. Just as a conductor directs and controls a symphony orchestra, similarly, genes are master molecules that control the overall activities in our bodies. But genes do not act alone. They act in response to a stimulus or an environment, which could be either external or internal. This implies that all genetic activity is subject to gene-environment interaction, that is, genes act when they are exposed to a certain specific environmental factor. This does not mean that all the genes in a human cell become active when exposed to certain stimuli. In that event, there would be a total discordance and functional failure in the human body. To avert such a catastrophe, nature has so evolved that only a small fraction of genes in a given cell are active. A certain set of genes are active in a particular cell type and are responsible for the specific properties of that cell type. In other words, even though there are a large number of genes in a human cell, only a small fraction of these genes are active in a given cell. Different genes are active in different cells, resulting in cells with different properties. For example, haemoglobin genes are active in blood cells but not in nerve cells, and genes for melanin synthesis are active in the skin cells but not in the liver cells. Although, so far, it is not very clear why a certain gene is active whereas another gene is non-active, or shut off in a cell type, it seems highly likely that specific gene-environment interactions play a critical role in selective 'activation' or 'suppression' of a specific gene.

COMPOSITION OF A GENE

Each gene consists of a very long molecule called deoxyribonucleic acid or DNA. DNA is made up of many small subunits called nucleotides. There are four kinds of nucleotides known, each containing a different nitrogenous base in the subunit: two purines, adenine (A), and guanine (G); and two pyrimidines, thymine (T), and cytosine (C). These four letters, A, G, T, and C constitute the genetic dictionary, and their combinations and *sequences* encode all the genetic information in all forms of life. A single gene may contain 600 to several thousands of the nucleotide units. More importantly, it is the sequence of subunits in a DNA molecule which is characteristic of a particular gene, and these sequences differ from one gene to another. In other words, the differences between genes lie in the precise sequence of nucleotides, which confers on each gene the unique property to specify its genetic code.

The four subunits are joined together in long chains, and the DNA molecule consists of two such long chains wound around each other in a double helix (Fig. 3.1A). The order in which the subunits are arranged in one chain dictates the arrangement of subunits in the other chain. For example, whenever one chain contains an A subunit, the other chain contains a T subunit at the corresponding place. Likewise, whenever a G subunit is located on one chain, a C subunit is located in the corresponding position in the other chain. This rule of A pairing with T, and G pairing with C is based on the chemical properties of these subunits. Thus, A and T form a complementary pair, and G and C form another complementary pair, and this built-in complementarity of AT and GC pairs gives the DNA molecule a highly precise and specific profile necessary for the transmission of genetic material from one parent cell to its daughter cells in an individual or to the next generation.

GENES IN CELL DIVISION

When a cell divides, it first produces a copy of all the chromosomal material and thus provides a complete

A. PARENTAL DOUBLE HELIX

B. REPLICATION OF NEW DAUGHTER DUPLEXES

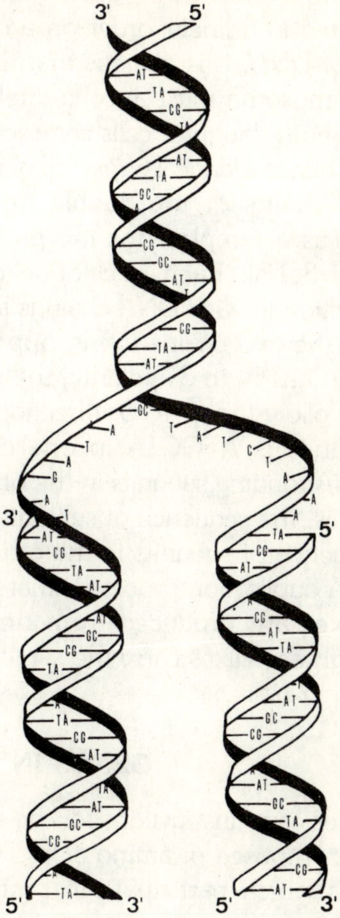

Fig. 3.1 The DNA double helix (A) and duplication of a parental DNA duplex into two daughter duplexes (B). During the duplication process, the two parental strands separate, and while this is happening, each strand acts as a template on which a new DNA strand is synthesized. At the end of this process, two identical DNA duplexes are produced from a single DNA duplex. The base pairing in the DNA duplex is very specific: A (adenine) always pairs with T (thymine), and G (guanine) with C (cytosine).

chromosome set to each daughter cell. Since genes are located in a linear order on a chromosome, and are made up of DNA, it is obvious that the DNA double helix in each chromosome must also be duplicated before cell division so that both daughter cells can receive identical copies of DNA, and hence identical copies of genes. During DNA duplication, two chains of the double helix unwind and each chain acts as a template for the production of the second chain (Fig. 3.1B). Each nucleotide chain has polarity, and the direction in each DNA chain is indicated by 5′ to 3′ notation, and the two chains run in opposite direction, that is, if one chain has 5′ to 3′ polarity, the second complementary chain will follow the 3′ to 5′ direction. Further, if the sequence of subunits is ATGCTA in one chain, then the sequence of corresponding subunits in the other chain would be TACGAT, that is, the sequence of subunits in one chain determines the sequence of subunits in the other chain. The end result of a DNA duplication process is that two identical daughter double helixes are produced from one mother double helix; the daughter helixes carry the same sequence of subunits as the mother helix.

GENES IN ACTION

Genes carry instructions for the synthesis of proteins. Proteins are composed of amino acids. There are 20 different amino acids which participate in protein synthesis in our bodies. Protein molecules may consist of several hundred to several thousand amino acids. There are only four subunits in the DNA molecule, A, T, G, C, known as four letters of the genetic code, and these must code for the 20 different amino acids. The genetic code has been deciphered; it is a three-letter (triplet) code. Since we have four letters, A,T,G and C, and the code is triplet, it is possible to have 64 (4^3) three-letter code words. Thus, for example, AGA, GAA, and AAG are three different code words. The 64 code words are more than sufficient to code for the 20 amino acids required for protein synthesis. It is apparent that there is an excess of 44 code words. Therefore, it is not surprising that some of the amino acids are specified by more than one code word. Moreover, some code words have additional functions, particularly those that code for 'start' and 'stop' signals for protein synthesis.

The genes do not directly give instructions to amino acids to line up in a certain sequence so as to produce a protein molecule, but do so through an intermediary molecule known as messenger ribonucleic acid (mRNA). The first phase of the transmittance of the genetic code takes place when genetic messages are passed on from DNA to RNA molecules. The DNA and RNA molecules are similar in their subunit composition except for one subuniit T, which is replaced in the RNA by subunit U (uracil), and in terms of pairing behaviour, U pairs with A. That means when an RNA molecule is produced on a DNA template, it also carries the complementary subunits A, G, and C, but not T, which is substituted by U (Fig. 3.2). Thus, a code word CAT from the DNA molecule is transcribed as a GUA triplet in the mRNA, and GCT as CGA, and so on. The triplet GUA specifies the amino acid valine, whereas CGA is the code word for the amino acid arginine. As mentioned earlier, there is more than one code word for each of several amino acids. Thus amino acid valine is prescribed not only by the triplet GUA, but also by GUC, GUG, and GUU; arginine is also designated by additional triplets CGC, CGG, AGA, and AGG. Other amino acids are designated by variable numbers (2-6) of triplets. Three amino acids are transcribed by one triplet each: tryptophane by UGG, glutamic acid by GAG, and methionine by AUG, and these also happen to be the start signal for protein synthesis. Another three triplets UAA, UAG, and UGA signal the end of the message. The 64 RNA triplets specifying for 20 different amino acids are shown in Table 3.1.

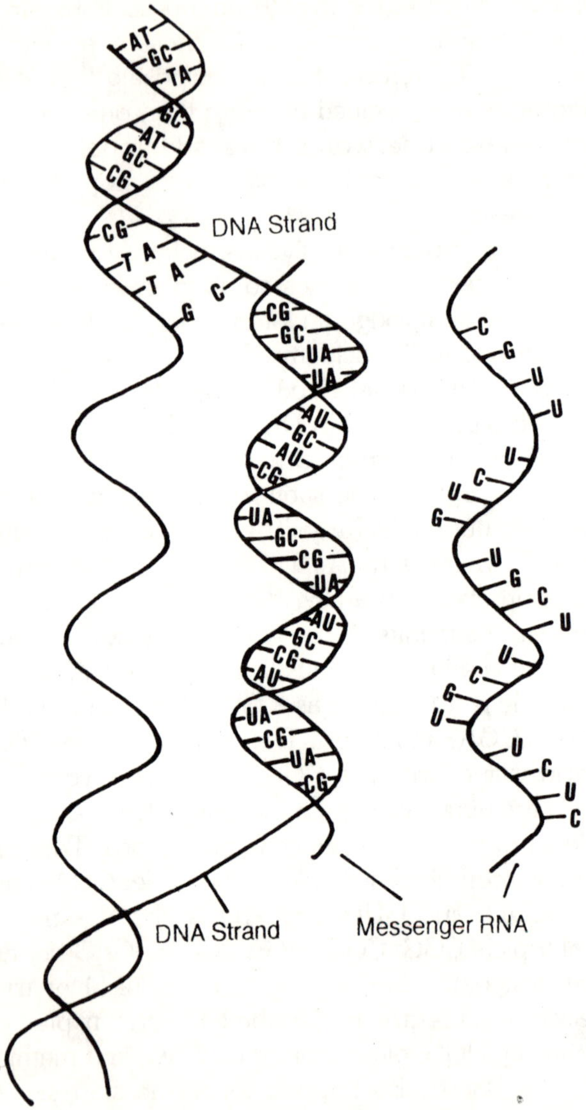

Fig. 3.2 **Production of messenger RNA (mRNA) molecule on a DNA template. The DNA and RNA have similar bases, except for one: thymine (T) in DNA is replaced by uracil (U) in the RNA.**

Table 3.1 The genetic code (64 triplets) arranged according to the number of code words specifying an amino acid

Triplet codon	*Amino acid*	*Triplet codon*	*Amino acid*
AUG	Methionine	AUU	Isoleucine
UGG	Tryptophane	AUC	Isoleucine
GAA	Glutamic acid	AUA	Isoleucine
GAG	Glutamic acid	UAA	End of message
UUU	Phenylalanine	UAG	End of message
UUC	Phenylalanine	UGA	End of message
UGU	Cysteine	GCC	Alanine
UGC	Cysteine	GCU	Alanine
AAA	Lysine	GCA	Alanine
AAG	Lysine	GCG	Alanine
AAU	Asparagine	GGU	Glycine
AAC	Asparagine	GGC	Glycine
GAU	Aspartic acid	GGA	Glycine
GAC	Aspartic acid	GGG	Glycine
CAA	Glutamine	ACU	Threonine
CAG	Glutamine	ACC	Threonine
CAU	Histidine	ACA	Threonine
CAC	Histidine	ACG	Threonine

(*cont'd.*)

Triplet codon	*Amino acid*	*Triplet codon*	*Amino acid*
UAU	Tyrosine	CCC	Proline
UAC	Tyrosine	CCA	Proline
CCU	Proline	CGA	Arginine
CCG	Proline	CGG	Arginine
GUC	Valine	AGA	Arginine
GUG	Valine	AGG	Arginine
GUU	Valine	CGC	Arginine
GUA	Valine	CGU	Arginine
UUA	Leucine		
UUG	Leucine		
CUU	Leucine		
CUC	Leucine		
CUA	Leucine		
CUG	Leucine		
UCU	Serine		
UCC	Serine		
UCA	Serine		
UCG	Serine		
AGU	Serine		
AGC	Serine		

A fascinating sequence of events occurs during protein synthesis. A DNA template is transcribed onto an mRNA molecule. This mRNA molecule carries the message from the nucleus to the cytoplasm. In addition to mRNA, two other types of RNAs, ribosomal RNA (rRNA), and transfer RNA (tRNA), required for protein synthesis, are also transcribed on the DNA templates, and move on to the cytoplasm where protein synthesis occurs. Specific amino acids are lined up by the tRNAs at the protein-manufacturing factory, the ribosomes, and, in the presence of mRNA carrying a specific coded message in triplets, the amino acids are guided by tRNAs in the specific sequence for the building of a protein molecule. The sequence of amino acids in a protein gives the protein its unique properties. Therefore, each gene, through its mRNA, codes for a specific protein.

Gene expression is controlled by controlling regions of DNA, the so-called *regulatory genes*, which are located either next to the structural genes or at sites distant from these genes. Regulatory genes either prevent, or, in some cases, stimulate the production of proteins. Regulatory genes are involved in the control of all life processes, including cell reproduction and cell differentiation. Therefore, smooth and unimpaired regulatory gene function is a prerequisite for the existence of a healthy organ. What would happen in case of an impairment of the regulatory gene function? It seems logical that when the regulatory genes lose control over cell reproduction and cell differentiation, there would be a lack of order in form and function, which may lead to the origin of cancer. Why does a regulatory gene lose its power of control? This could be due to an impairment or mutation of a regulatory gene, or of some other genes affecting the functioning of the control gene.

MUTATION

Mutation can be defined as a heritable change or alteration in the genetic material (DNA). Mutations may occur either at the chromosomal level through loss, addition, or rearrangement of chromosomes, or at a gene level. In general, chromosomal loss, addition, or rearrangement would lead to loss or impairment of one function or perhaps many specific gene functions. Mutations at a gene level, known as point mutation, may also lead to loss or impairment of a gene function. At the level of DNA, one type of mutation which is fairly well understood involves substitution of a certain subunit or subunits in the genetic code of a gene. For example, the triplet CAT codes for the amino acid valine through its mRNA triplet GUA. Now, if the letter G is substituted for the letter C, then the DNA triplet would read GAT rather than CAT. This new triplet GAT would translate into the mRNA triplet CUA, so that leucine would be specified instead of valine. Thus a mutation in the DNA consisting of a substitution of a single letter C by G alters the protein function. Even a single change in the genetic code may prevent the protein from functioning normally, or, in some cases, from functioning at all. Sometimes, this alteration of proteins resulting from a mutation may lead to a change in the behaviour of a cell, or be the cause of its death.

In the present context the mutation concept is important for our discussion because at least in some cases a mutation or mutations in a regulatory gene or genes function may lead to loss of control over cell reproduction and/or cell differentiation and thus may create a cancer cell. Mutations can be caused by diverse agents such as X-rays, ultraviolet rays, and many chemicals (see Chapters 9 and 10). Many studies conducted on a variety of different plant and animal test systems have shown that the agents which cause mutations may also be involved in the origin of cancer. This would suggest that the environmental mutagens may cause cancer by inducing mutations in the genetic material, very likely in the regulatory genes.

4

The Cell Cycle and Cancer

THE FOUR PERIODS OF THE CELL CYCLE

Cell division is an integral part of the cell cycle. Before a cell divides, it must undergo a series of preparations, which take a much longer time than the actual cell division itself. The entire period consisting of preparations before the division, and during division itself, constitutes a cell cycle or cell generation time. The cell cycle can be divided into four discrete periods (Fig. 4.1). These are designated as: a pre-synthetic period (G1), followed by a DNA synthetic period (S), the post-DNA synthetic period (G2), and division or mitosis period (D or M). Here, G1 denotes the interval between the initiation of the cell cycle and the onset of chromosomal DNA synthesis. In the G1 period the cell must primarily prepare its machinery for enzymes and substrates required for DNA replication. The G1 period is followed by the S period during which DNA synthesis occurs. The interval between the end of DNA synthesis and the beginning of cell division is the G2 period. The interval during which the cell divides is known as the D or M period. These four periods are well coordinated in a normal individual. However, each cell type divides at a specific rate and, therefore, differential growth rates of different cell types reflect the variation in their cell generation time.

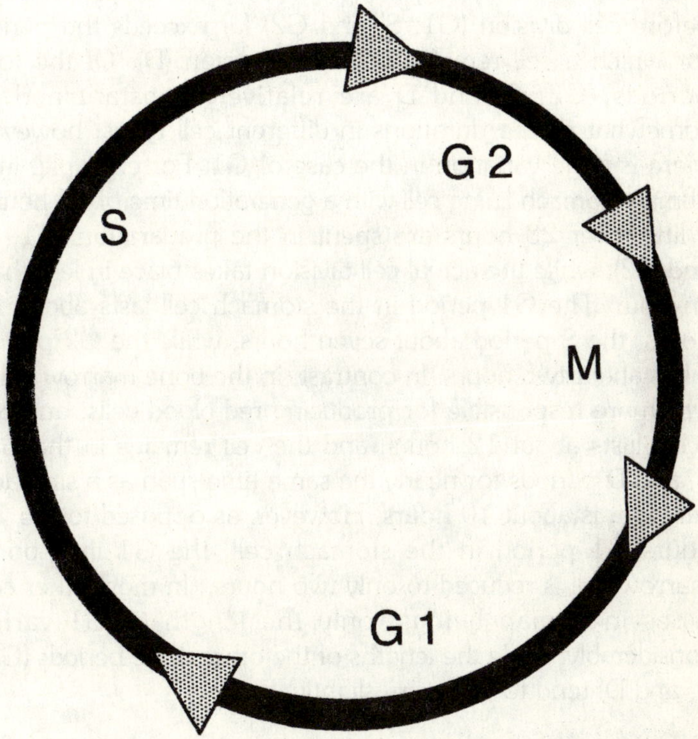

Fig. 4.1 The cell cycle consists of four periods: the G1, G2, S, and M or D. During the G1 and G2 periods, the cell prepares the enzymatic machinery for the division of a cell. DNA synthesis occurs during the S period, while actual cell division occurs during the D or M period. Other than the G1 period, the lengths of the remaining periods in the cell cycle, that is, G2, S, and M, are less variable.

VARIABLE AND CONSTANT COMPONENTS OF THE CELL CYCLE

Normal Cell

The cell generation time varies in different cell types. However, in all cell types the time spent on preparation before cell division (G1, S, and G2) far exceeds the period for which a cell remains in actual division (D). Of the four periods, G2, S, and D are relatively constant and of somewhat similar durations in different cell types; however, there is large variation in the case of G1. For example, in a human stomach lining cell with a generation time of 24 hours, a little over 23 hours are spent in the preparation (G1, S, and G2), while the actual cell division takes place in less than an hour. The G1 period in the stomach cell lasts about 14 hours, the S period about seven hours, while the G2 period takes about two hours. In contrast, in the bone marrow cells, which are responsible for producing red blood cells, one cell cycle lasts about 12 hours, and the cell remains in the G2, S, and D periods for nearly the same time span as a stomach cell, that is about 10 hours. However, as opposed to the 14 hours G1 period in the stomach cell, the G1 in a bone marrow cell is reduced to only two hours. In most other cell types in human beings, only the length of G1 varies considerably, while the lengths of the other three periods (G2, S, and D) tend to vary very slightly.

Cancer Cell

The cell cycle of a cancer cell, as in a normal cell, is also subdivided into the same four periods, that is, G1, G2, S, and D. The length of the interval of the different periods is nearly the same: for example, in the case of a normal stomach lining cell with a generation time of 24 hours, or that of a leukaemic (cancer) cell with a cell cycle of, again,

24 hours. Therefore, it would appear that a normal growing cell and a cancer cell cannot be distinguished from one another as far as the periods of the cell cycle are concerned. If the normal cell and the cancer cell are both indistinguishable in terms of the four periods (G1, S, G2, and D) in their cell cycles, then in what way can we differentiate the two? Does the cancer cell differ from its normal counterpart cell in any specific way when the different periods of the cell cycle are examined individually? We shall find out answers to these questions in the following sections.

THE CELL DIVISION

Normal Cell

Let us first examine the cell division or the D period of a normal cell, and then compare it to the D period of a cancer cell. The D period is divided into the following phases: interphase, prophase, metaphase, anaphase and telophase. During interphase (Fig. 4.2a) the chromosomal DNA synthesis (S period) and specific types of RNA and proteins are synthesized (G2 period), as the nucleus of the cell prepares to divide. The reticular network in the nucleus resolves itself into visible chromosomes and the cell enters the prophase. During prophase the chromosomes are already duplicated and appear as long-drawn double threads (Fig. 4.2b). At least three distinct events occur during prophase: (a) the chromosomes shorten considerably in length and each chromosome appears double; (b) the nucleoli gradually shrink and fade away; and (c) the nuclear membrane breaks apart and disappears. Prophase is followed by metaphase during which the visibly double chromosomes attain the maximum contraction and move to the centre of a cell where they are arranged on the equatorial plate. The chromosomes are held in this position by a spindle apparatus (Fig. 4.2c). During the late metaphase, each chromosome appears longitudinally split

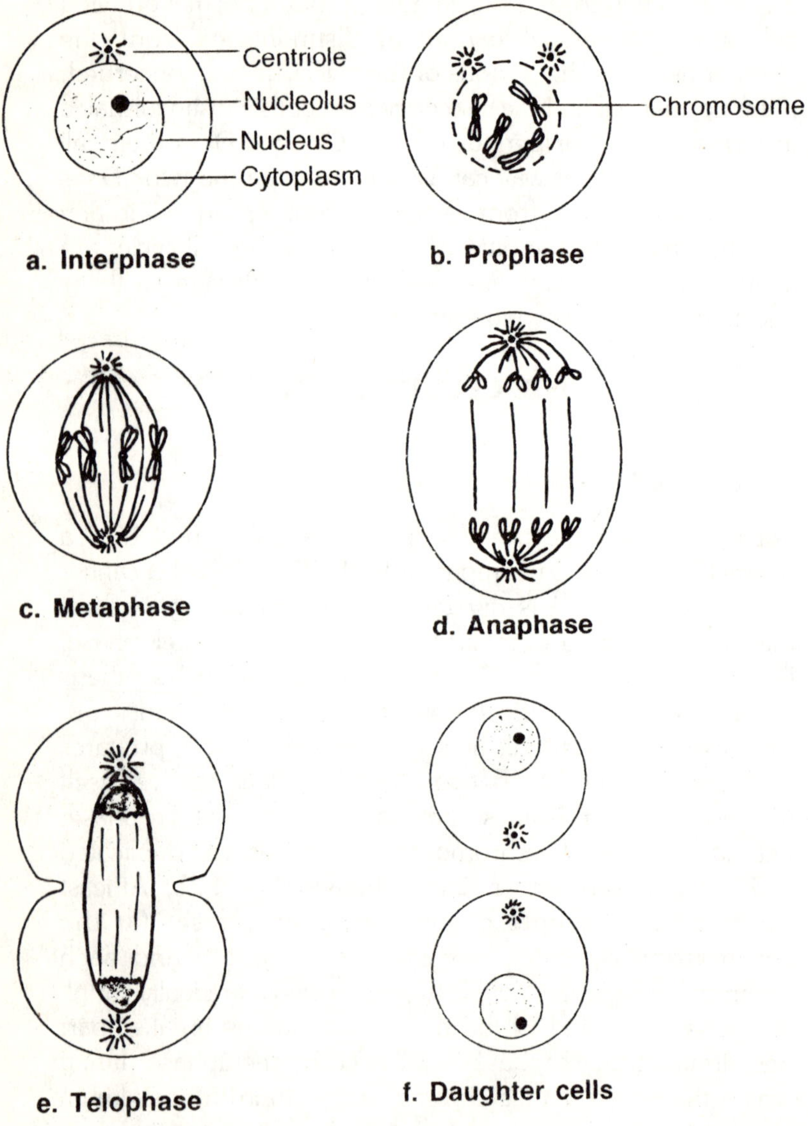

Fig. 4.2 **Stages of cell division. When a body cell divides by mitosis, it gives rise to two identical cells, which carry the same chromosome number as the parental cells.**

into half-chromosomes (chromatids) along its entire length, including the region of the spindle attachment (centromere). Metaphase is followed by anaphase during which the longitudinally split chromosomes separate and move towards the poles of the cell, and it appears as if the half-chromosomes are drawn away from the centre of the cell by the contraction of the spindle apparatus (Fig. 4.2d). When the chromosome movement is completed, the cell enters telophase, the last phase of the D period. During telophase the chromosomes begin to lose their identity and the network character of the metabolic nucleus, the nuclear membrane and the nucleoli begin to develop (Fig. 4.2e). While these events are progressing, the cell itself divides into two daughter cells during telophase. The end result of a mitotic division is that, by this process, a cell gives rise to two daughter cells (Fig. 4.2f) having an identical set of chromosomes with an identical set of genes. Therefore, cell division provides a precise means of transmitting the identical genetic information to the descendants of a single cell.

Cell division is the principal component of growth, whether it is normal tissue or a cancerous tissue, and provides means for the replacement of worn or dead cells in a living organism. In a normal individual the cells reproduce to perform the necessary functions, and there is a delicate balance between cell reproduction and cell death. This process is so precisely regulated in a normal tissue that at a given time there is a constant number of functional cells.

Cancer Cell

The cancer cell also undergoes all the five phases of cell division (interphase, prophase, metaphase, anaphase and telophase) and the duration of all these phases is nearly the same as compared to its counterpart normal cell type from which it is derived. Therefore, it would appear that the cancer cell may not have a serious defect in any one of the cell division phases, but may have a defect in the G1, S, or G2 periods of the cell cycle. The durations of the S and the G2 periods in a cancer cell tend to vary very little when compared to its normal counterpart cell type. This leaves the G1 period as a possible source of defect in a cancer cell. It is well known that cancer cells are a rapidly proliferating population of cells which neither mature into normal form nor participate in the replacement of normal cells lost due to one cause or another. Therefore, the cancer cells serve practically no useful cellular function whatsoever. How can a defect in the G1 period of the cell account for the proliferative and functionless posture of a cancer cell? Before we answer this question, let us first examine the cell division rates and the cell cycles in some normal human cell types, and determine how these rates might be related to the G1 period.

G1 PERIOD AND CELL PROLIFERATION

Normal Cell

In the mammalian cells, the S phase lasts for about 6-8 hours, the G2 period for 2-6 hours, and the D phase for about 1 hour, but there is considerable variation in the duration of G1 in different cell types. It is an interesting phenomenon that the length of the G1 period is the most variable as compared to the remaining three periods of the cell cycle. In other words, the rates of cell division in different cell types may be, to a large extent, determined by the regulation of the G1 interval. For example, in the earliest stages of human embryo development the cells divide very rapidly, and consequently, may have a virtually zero G1 interval, while the nerve cells and some muscle cells, which do not divide in an adult human being, may be permanently arrested in the G1 period. A very large number of cell types in an adult human fall between these two extremes of the G1 period. For example, in the bone marrow cells, which are responsible for producing red blood cells, one cell cycle lasts for about 12 hours, of which the length of the G1 period is approximately 2 hours, whereas a cell cycle in a stomach lining cell lasts for almost 24 hours, with a G1 period of 14 hours. Consequently, the cell cycle rate in both these cell types is relativlely high. On the other hand, the cells of the colon and the skin may divide only once every several days, while the liver cell may divide once in several months, and there seems to be a corresponding increase in the length of the G1 period ranging from hundreds of hours in colon and skin to thousands of hours for the liver cells. Therefore, regulation of the cell reproduction, depending upon the intrinsic demands of a specific human tissue, may be achieved by holding a cell for an appropriate time in the G1 period. Although the molecular mechanisms for retaining a cell in the G1 period are not well understood, it is probable that the regulatory mechanisms may in some way affect some activity of the cell in the G1 period before the cell enters the S period or beginning of the DNA replication in a specific cell type.

Cancer Cell

Based on the proliferative posture of a cancer cell, it might appear (a) that the defect in the G1 period of a cancer may be complete, that is, the cancer cell would divide continuously without being retained in the G1 period or (b) that the defect in the G1 period may be partial, so that the retention period in G1 is considerably reduced, and, as a result, the cancer cell would appear to divide at a relatively faster rate as compared to its normal counterpart cell type. The first possibility that the defect in the G1 period is complete does not appear to be tenable in cancer, since almost all types of cancer cells go through the G1 phase, however variable. It has been observed that different types of cancer cells do not divide at similar rates. For example, blood cells, skin cells, and liver cells do not divide at the same rate, but rather at cell division rates related to their tissue of origin. In many cases, the cell cycles of the cancer cells are thought to be shorter than the cell cycles of their normal counterpart cell types, implying that the cancer cells may be retained in the G1 interval for a relatively shorter period than their normal counterpart, and, consequently, the cancer cells undergo cell division more frequently. On the other hand, in some cases, the cell cycle may be longer in the cancer cells as compared to their cell type of origin. Certain cancers of the blood (leukaemias) and liver (hepatomas) have cell cycles longer than their normal counterpart cells. Obviously, in these cases, the G1 interval of their cell cycles would be longer as compared to the normal cells from which they are derived. Clearly, the defect in the G1 period is not complete, but seems to be partial, as, in most cases, the cancer cells are retained in the G1 period for a certain time, this interval being dependent upon the degree of defect in the G1 period.

NORMAL CELLS BEHAVE LIKE CANCER CELLS DURING REGENERATION

Another important aspect of the living cells is their flexibility in the rate of cell division. Under normal conditions, there is a balance between cell reproduction and cell death. The cells have a limited life span, and following the completion of this life span they die. For example, the life span of a red blood cell is about 120 days, while the life span of cells lining the intestine may be one or two days. When these cells, and for that matter other cell types, die, they are promptly replaced by cell reproduction. Further, most normal cells have a built-in flexibility to replace their kind at an accelerated rate when such cells are lost or damaged due to an accident. For example, excessive loss of blood leads to rapid reproduction of the blood-forming cells, and when the necessary number of blood cells have been formed, the cell reproduction stabilizes itself to a normal replacement rate. Similarly, when there is an injury to the skin (cuts, burns), the healing process occurs by an accelerated rate of cell reproduction in the deeper layers of the skin. In the same way, when a part of the liver is removed surgically, the remaining liver cells regenerate to the complete organ in a couple of weeks. This means that the process of regeneration is finely regulated in the normal cells, and after restoration of the necessary number of cells following an injury or operation, the cell reproduction again proceeds at rates characteristic of a cell type prior to the damage. During the regeneration process, the normal cells may temporarily behave like cancer cells as far as rapid proliferation is concerned, but the cell reproduction in a normal cell, unlike a cancer cell, is so well controlled that the start and the stop signals are recognized by the normal cell. Therefore, following regeneration of a tissue, normal growth and development are restored.

CONTINUOUS AND UNCONTROLLED CELL REPRODUCTION IN CANCER CELLS

In many types of cancer cells, the rate of reproduction appears to be higher than that of their normal counterparts. However, there are exceptions. The abnormal cell reproduction rates in the cancer cells are probably due to a partial defect in the G1 period of the cell cycle, the rate of cell reproduction of a cancer cell being dependent on the cell type of its origin. Whatever the reproduction rates, all tissue-specific cancers eventually build up cell masses that far outnumber the normal cells in those tissues. Therefore, it is not the rate of cell reproduction or the length of the cell cycle *per se* only which is important to the cancer problem, but rather it is the inherent capacity of a cancer cell to undergo *continuous* and *uncontrolled* cell reproduction, and its inability to mature normally and perform useful functions. Since cancer cells are perpetually dividing the population of cells, the initial defect may be in the regulatory control over the step(s) leading to chromosomal DNA synthesis.

5

Cell Differentiation and Cancer

Cell growth and differentiation constitute the two most important processes for the development of multicellular organisms. The life of a new human begins when a male's sperm nucleus fuses with a female's egg nucleus following an act of fertilization. The sperm and the egg nuclei carry 23 chromosomes each. As a result, in the normal human body, each cell contains 23 pairs of chromosomes, of which there is one pair of sex chromosomes; the male has an XY pair, while the female carries an XX pair. A male produces two kinds of gametes (the sperms): one half of these carry the X chromosome, the other half contain the Y chromosome. On the other hand, the female produces only one kind of gamete (the egg): each carries only one X chromosome. When sex cells are formed in a male or a female, the number of chromosomes in these cells is reduced to one half (23 chromosomes). The sex of a child is determined when an X- or Y-carrying sperm nucleus fuses with an X-carrying egg. Therefore, fertilization is an important event, since it restores the number of chromosomes to 46, which is characteristic of normal human body cells. In other words, the body cells of a human have one set of chromosomes contributed by each parent.

GROWTH AND DIFFERENTIATION IN THE HUMAN EMBRYO AND AN ADULT

At the time of fertilization the human egg weighs about one millionth of a gram ($1x10^{-6}$ gram) , whereas the sperm weighs even less ($5x10^{-9}$ gram). At birth, an average human baby weighs around 7 pounds (3200 grams); this represents an increase of about one billion times during the nine-month prenatal (before birth) period. The increase in the mass of a human embryo occurs as a result of cell reproduction and cell enlargement. At birth, the new born baby is not simply a haphazard mass of cells, but has a definite shape and form. Obviously, the growth of the embryo has been accompanied by a process called *differentiation*, which involves the formation of cells specialized for specific functions, such as nerve cells, heart cells, liver cells, stomach cells, lung cells, eye cells, kidney cells and muscle cells.

Following fertilization, the resultant zygote undergoes its first cell division after 24 hours. This is followed by cell proliferation over the next few days, producing a mass of a few dozen cells which appear identical to each other. In due course of time a number of growth centres arise amongst the embryonal cells. Subsequently, rapid cell production occurs in each growth centre, however, at different rates and times, resulting in a change of shape. These growth centres are coordinated to produce specialized forms and structures. For example, in a human embryo the head and neck increase in size rapidly during the early period of embryonal development, and the arms grow at a faster rate than the legs, but the trunk develops at a more or less steady rate until maturity. As specialization of the structure and the form proceeds, different cells differentiate into tissues and organs, thus giving the growing foetus its characteristic form, and hence distinguishing one individual from another. By birth a human baby consists of about 5 trillion (5×10^{12}) cells, representing 100 or more cell types. From birth through adolescence to adulthood, cell division continues in many groups of cells at rates intrinsic for each cell type. The body of an adult human with average height and weight may finally consist of some 100 trillion (10^{14}) cells. The important fact is that trillions of cells are derived from the original single cell – the zygote. Clearly, the zygote has the blueprint for the orderly development of all tissues and organs of an individual, whether female or male.

DIFFERENTIATION: A HERITABLE AND WELL-COORDINATED PROCESS

From the time of fertilization, through subsequent foetal development, up to the completion of the mature individual, the rates of cell reproduction in different tissues are regulated precisely. For example, the precursors of red blood cells in the bone marrow continue to undergo cell reproduction at a specific rate throughout the life of an individual. In contrast, the nerve cells continue to reproduce during the prenatal stage, but a complete cessation of cell reproduction occurs as soon as the necessary number has been produced; after birth there is virtually no further cell division in the nerve cells. That means, in a normal individual, the processes of cell reproduction and cell differentiation are perfectly coordinated and well regulated, so that there is normal functioning of different tissues. In the cancerous tissue, on the other hand, such perfect coordination between cell reproduction and differentiation is lacking, and the cancer cells do not mature to perform any useful function. The cancer cells have an altered genetic programme resulting from defective genes which steer the cancer cells towards uncontrolled growth, poor differentiation, and invasive behaviour.

In addition to cell reproduction and differentiation, cell death is also involved in maintaining a delicate balance for the development of multicellular organisms. Naturally occurring cell death is essential for tissue remodelling, for the production of body structures (such as skin and hair), and for cell replacement. With the exception of nerve cells and certain muscle cells, which do not undergo cell reproduction in the adult, most normal cell types in different tissues and organs continue to reproduce and differentiate in order to replace worn-out or dead cells. Therefore, each cell type has a reservoir of stem cells which undergo reproduction. It would appear that of the two products of cell division, one daughter cell contributes to the stem cell pool, whereas the second daughter cell undergoes further differentiation, finally maturing to produce functional proteins characteristic of a specific cell type. For example, fully mature red blood cells contain the protein haemoglobin, which gives blood its characteristic red colour and transports oxygen to different tissues of the body. The mature pancreatic cells produce the hormone insulin which breaks down sugar in the body. In normal tissues, there exists a balance among the stem cell pool, the differentiated cell pool, and the mature cell pool (Fig. 5.1A). The fully differentiated and mature cells in a tissue do not undergo further cell reproduction, and after the completion of their life spans, they die.

CLONAL ORIGIN OF CANCER

Experimental evidence suggests that most human cancers are clonal in origin, that is, they arise from a single defective cell. From this single cell populations of cancer cells are produced by division and growth, of which a proportion of cells may be retained as stem cells for renewal, due to cell loss or death, and for generating malignant tumour masses. Depending upon the cell type, cancer cells may be arrested at some stage in the differentiation pathway (for example, laeukaemia, melanoma), or they may undergo a degree of differentiation and maturation (for example, solid tumours). In other words, the tumour cells also appear to have a reservoir of stem cells and may undergo some differentiation and maturation, as well as cell death. In this respect, cancer cells may be kinetically active in growth and differentiation, as are the normal cells. However, the delicate balance between cell birth and cell death is disturbed in the cancer cells, as cell birth exceeds cell death and this results in tumour expansion. Cell loss or

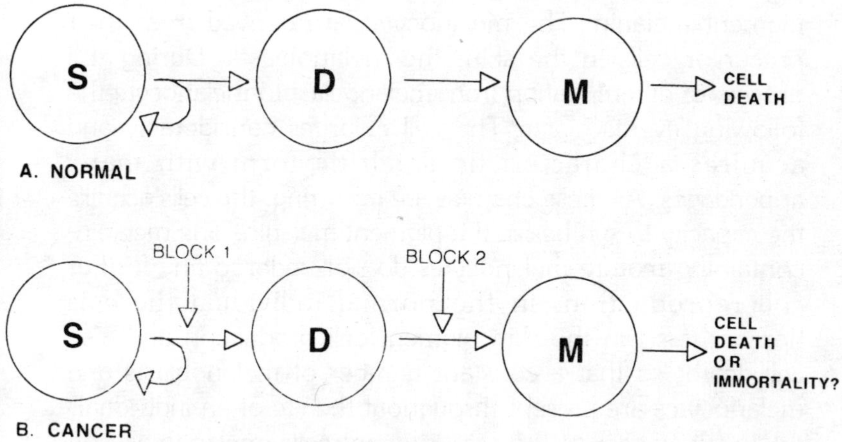

Fig. 5.1 Stages of cell differentiation. A: In normal cell differentiation, a stem cell divides and, of the two products of cell division, one is returned to the stem pool (S), while the second daughter cell undergoes differentiation (D) and maturation (M), and finally programmed cell death. B: By contrast, the cancer cells remain undifferentiated or undergo incomplete or aberrant cell differentiation. These states result from blocks at any stage of differentiation: block 1 would result in cumulation of cells in the stem or precursor pool (S), while block 2 would lead to cumulation of cells in the differentiated pool (D). Cancer cells rarely undergo maturation, and the cell death programme is disturbed.

cell death in tumours may be due to terminal differentiation, inadequate nutrition, and aberrant chromosomes (aneuploidy) in mitosis. As mentioned earlier, in some cancers the cells remain undifferentiated or incompletely differentiated, and these cells do not mature (Fig. 5.1B). Two types of cancers, melanoma and leukaemia, are now presented below as examples of defects in cell differentiation.

Melanoma

The skin of a normal individual contains a large number of pigment cells, the melanocytes. These contain the dark pigment melanin. The melanocytes are derived from their precursor cells in the skin, the melanoblasts. During the process of differentiation from melanoblast to melanocyte the following events occur. The cell enlarges considerably and acquires a characteristic dendritic form with many appendages. As these changes are occurring, the cells acquire the capacity to synthesize the pigment melanin. The melanin-containing mature melanocytes do not undergo any further cell reproduction. In the normal individual there is homoeostasis in the skin pigment cell production and also cell death, so that a constant number of melanoblasts and melanocytes are present throughout the life of an individual.

In the cancer of the skin pigment cells (melanomas), on the other hand, the melanoblasts generally do not differentiate, so that a greater abundance of useless melanoblast-like cells are produced which crowd out the normal melanoblasts and interfere with the normal functioning of the skin pigment cells. The incidence of melanoma is relatively higher in the white-skinned races as compared to dark-skinned races. This is related to the fact that the dark skin with a uniform distribution of melanin is far more efficient than the light skin in screening out the carcinogenic ultraviolet radiation. Consistent with this observation is the fact that albinos, who have a normal number of melanocytes but incapable of producing the dark pigment melanin, are particularly susceptible to the development of skin cancer when exposed to strong sunlight.

Leukaemia

There are different kinds of cancer of the blood cells (leukaemias) which afflict children and young adults. The normal functioning of the blood cells is carried out by various kinds of mature blood cells, such as red blood cells (erythrocytes), and the white blood cells (leucocytes or lymphocytes). In leukaemias there is a defect in the differentiation of blood stem cells from the bone marrow or the lymphoid tissue; the defect is predominantly in those involved in the differentiation of white blood cells. For example, in certain kinds of leukaemias there is a defect in the bone marrow leucocyte maturation. The immature white blood cells (lymphocytes) are produced in great excess and interfere with the normal functioning of the blood. In a normal individual the mature lymphocytes acquire the ability to defend the individual against infection by bacteria and viruses. On the other hand, in the leukaemic patients, the useless lymphocytes lack the capacity to defend the individual against infection. The abnormal lymphocytes infiltrate the bone marrow, the lymphoid and other organs. This is a process that eventually leads to deficiencies of normal blood cells as well as cells involved in the immune mechanisms of an individual.

Clearly then, the process of cell differentiation is extremely crucial for the characteristic development of different forms and structures in a normal individual. Cell differentiation not only occurs during embryonic development, but also continues throughout the life of an individual. The differentiated normal cells, upon reaching maturity, perform specialized functions necessary for the well-being of an individual. The cancer cells, on the other hand, may not undergo normal processes of differentiation and, to a large extent, remain incompletely differentiated, and, consequently, do not mature to perform any useful function. Instead, the cancer cells crowd out the normal cells, interfere with normal functions, and finally destroy the normal cells by their invasive behaviour.

6

Genes and Human Cancer

GENETIC AND ENVIRONMENTAL FACTORS

A worldwide survey of cancer incidence has revealed that there is variation in the human population with regard to the probabilities of occurrence of different cancers. The variation in the occurrence of cancer may be partly related to the environment, on the one hand, and to the genetic factors, on the other. It has also been observed that cancer incidence varies greatly from one country to another. For example: cancer of the liver is more common in Mozambique (Africa) than in Europe; Japan has a high incidence of stomach cancer as compared to the USA; cancer of the mouth is predominant in India; bladder cancer is more common in Egypt; whereas skin cancer is prevalent in countries with sunny climates. Therefore, when we consider the environmental influences on the incidence of cancer, we realize the tremendous impact of geography on human culture and habits. In some cases, specific environmental factors have been found to be associated with specific cancers; for example, aflotoxin with cancer of the liver, the type of diet with cancer of the stomach, ultraviolet radiation in sunlight with skin cancer, betel quid or 'pan' with cancer of the mouth, and cigarette smoking with lung cancer. Thus, international variation in the incidence of cancer depends at least in part on the environmental conditions prevalent in different countries. Aflotoxin is a frequent contaminant of foodstuff stored in hot and humid conditions, and may account for high incidence of liver cancer in Mozambique. Chewing 'pan' (containing betel nut, lime, and tobacco) is a local custom in India, and ingredients of the 'pan' seem to be associated with a high incidence of cancer of the mouth.

In addition to international variation in the incidence of cancer which appears largely due to environmental factors, variation also exists within the populations of each country. For example, within Mozambique, some individuals exposed to aflotoxin face, on this account, a high risk of liver cancer, whereas others, equally exposed, face a much lower risk. For instance, at an individual level, two sailors are exposed to bright sunlight day after day. One of them develops skin cancer, sometimes independently at different parts of the body, whereas the other escapes entirely. The risk of lung cancer is greatly increased in some individuals due to cigarette smoking, and much less so in others. One can cite many examples of this sort from everyday life. However, some exceptions may also be found. Sometimes, one twin may develop cancer and his comonozygotic twin may be spared. The underlying basis for variation between individuals who are exposed to the same environmental factors is largely determined by genetic factors. It is also interesting to note that there is also variation in the site-specific cancers between human females and males (Figs. 6.1, 6.2 and 6.3). The incidence of these cancers is partly dependent on the sex, the genotype, and the degree of exposure to the environmental factors. For example, in the United States of America, the lung cancer death rate has increased considerably in the males, as compared to the females between 1930 and 1990 (Figs. 6.1 and 6.2). According to the American Cancer Society's 1993 estimates, the incidence of breast cancer in the females would be 32 per cent, and

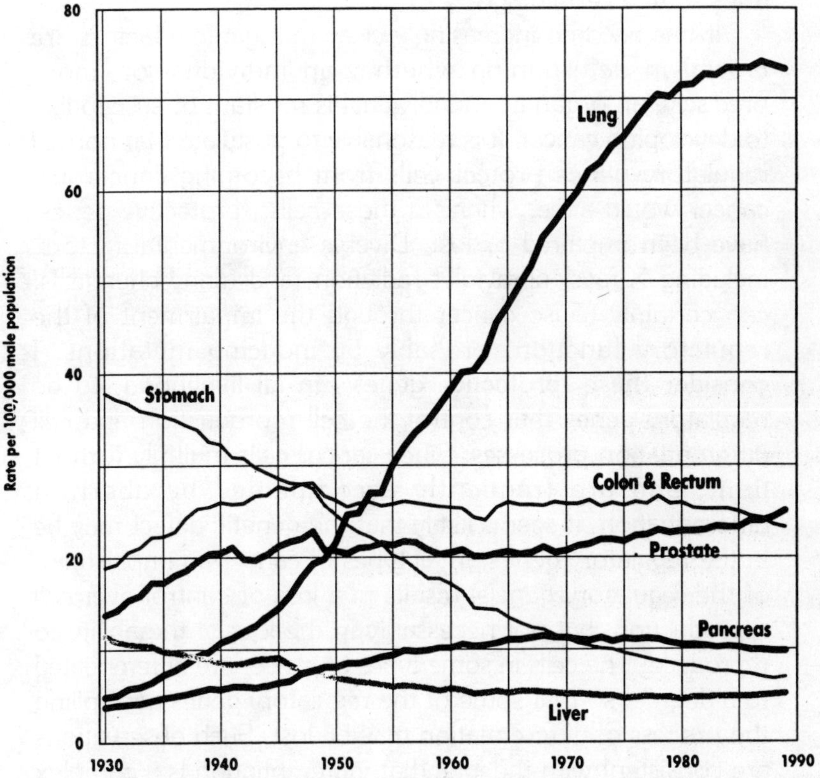

Fig. 6.1 Cancer death rates by site in American males over a 60-year period extending from 1930 to 1989 (reproduced with permission from the American Cancer Society, Atlanta, Georgia, USA).

that of prostate cancer in the males about 28 per cent, while the incidence of lung cancer in the males would be 17 per cent as compared to 12 per cent in the females (Fig. 6.3). However, in addition to the genetic predisposition, there is a large element called *chance*, which may be operative, at least, in most forms of cancer with respect to whether or not a person contracts cancer at all during his lifetime, or does so at a certain age.

It has become increasingly clear that genetic factors are crucial in determining whether an individual or, more precisely, an organ in an individual is resistant or susceptible to developing cancer. It is reasonable to postulate that normal regulatory genes protect cells from becoming cancerous; cancer would arise, when, in those cells, 'protective genes' have been impaired or lost. Diverse environmental factors, including X-rays, ultraviolet radiation, and many chemicals, can certainly cause cancer through the impairment of the regulatory function, probably by inducing mutations. I consider these 'protective genes', in all likelihood, to be regulatory genes that control the cell reproduction and cell differentiation processes. Since cancer cells multiply without limit, and are frequently accompanied by aberrant differentiation, it seems likely that the genetic defect may be in the regulatory genes. In all types of cancer an impairment of the regulatory gene(s) results in a loss of control over cell reproduction, but not necessarily in the loss of the ability to reproduce. The cells in some types of cancer are differentiated to a degree, so that some of the regulatory genes controlling the process of differentiation may be lost. Such observations are consistent with the idea that differentiation is a complex process and that a number of genes may be active in any given kind of tissue. It has been possible to demonstrate that most cancers originate from single somatic (body) cells, and since all the cell progeny of this cell (through a series of cell divisions) exhibit identical or very similar defects, cancer is believed to be a genetic disease.

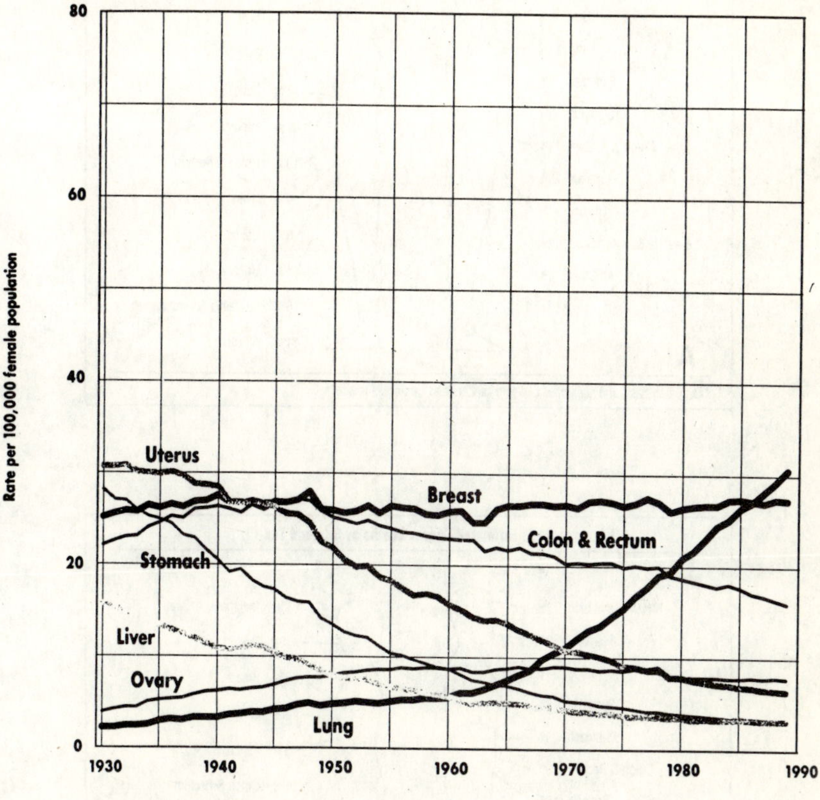

Fig. 6.2 Cancer death rates by site in American females over a 60-year period extending from 1930 to 1989 (reproduced with permission from the American Cancer Society, Atlanta, Georgia, USA).

It is necessary here to point out a difference in the meanings of the words 'genetic' and 'hereditary'. If a defect appears in a cell which is transmitted to its daughter cells and to further cell generations that can be traced to the

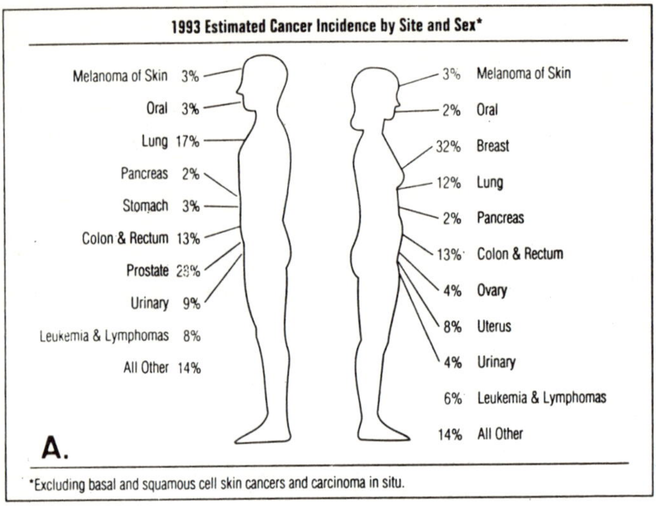

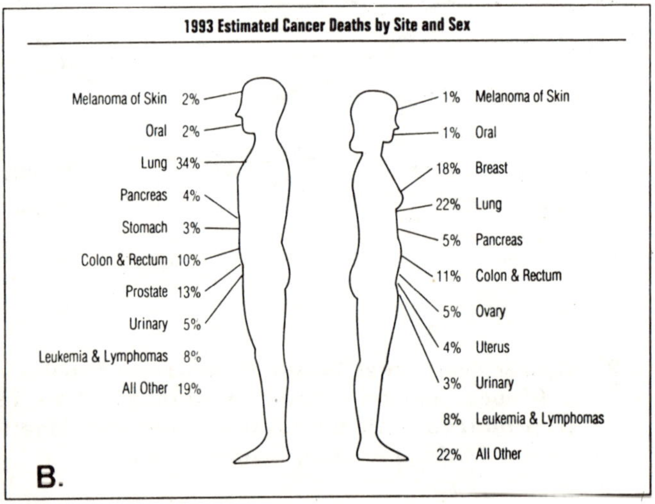

Fig. 6.3 Estimated cancer incidence (A) and deaths (B) by site and sex in the USA for the year 1993 (reproduced with permission from the American Cancer Society, Atlanta, Georgia, USA).

original defective cell, the condition can be considered 'genetic', in the sense that the defect is passed on without exception from one cell generation to the next. The term 'hereditary', however, is generally used to indicate that a trait in a plant, animal, or human is being passed on to the offspring or progeny. More precisely, it would often be the transmission, from parent to offspring, which would lead to tendency or susceptibility for a trait or defect to appear. Thus, cancer would always be genetic, in the sense just mentioned, and not always hereditary, and, if hereditary, it may be in various degrees.

GENETIC PREDISPOSITION TO CANCER

In this category several human cancers will be discussed, which exhibit genetic predisposition to the disease. In the familial cancers, the genetic susceptibility would be determined by the number of defective genes that are transmitted from parents to offspring.

Breast Cancer

Epidemiological studies worldwide have shown that the incidence of breast cancer is influenced by a number of factors. The risk factors for breast cancer in females include age, country of birth, socioeconomic class, marital status, race, degree of radiation to the chest, environmental effects, and hereditary predisposition. According to the American Cancer Society, there may be an estimated 182,000 (32 per cent) new cases of breast cancer among women in 1993 in the United States (Fig. 6.2). The incidence increases with advancing age and it is predicted that one out of every nine women will develop breast cancer by age 85 in the USA.

A large number of families with breast cancer histories have been investigated all over the world. These studies have indicated that genetic factors play an important role in the predisposition of women to breast cancer. Inherited influences are especially prominent in the premenopausal breast cancer. Female relatives of breast cancer probands are generally at a higher risk of developing breast cancer than female relatives of the normal probands. In one comprehensive study on mothers, grandmothers, aunts, and sisters, the sample women were divided into three groups: (1) women with diagnosed breast cancer; (2) women with some cancer other than breast cancer; and (3) women who had no breast cancer. Breast cancer occurred two to three times more frequently among relatives of the breast cancer probands as compared to women from groups 2 and 3. These results confirm that there is not only inherited predisposition to breast cancer but also that inherited predisposition is organ-specific.

Environmental factors, such as dietary fat, hormones, and perhaps viruses have also been implicated in the causation of breast cancer. Inasmuch as individuals differ in their genetic predisposition to breast (or perhaps any other) cancer, and also with respect to the aforementioned environmental factors, it is probably best to think of the causation resulting due to hereditary and environmental factors acting together; in some cases the environmental factors would be more important, and in others, the hereditary ones.

Recent advances in human genome mapping will be valuable in determining the site of not only normal genes, but also defective genes. In this regard, gene mapping studies have also been directed towards locating breast cancer susceptibility gene(s) in women, and according to molecular biologists Mary-Claire King, Donna Shattuck-Eidens, and Mark Skolnick, one such gene (BRCA-1) may be located on human chromosome 17.

Stomach Cancer

Extensive investigations have been carried out in search of evidence for genetic factors in stomach cancer. In general, stomach cancer occurs more frequently in the relatives of probands than in those of unrelated normal individuals used as controls, although in some studies the differences are not significant. Dietary factors, particularly nitrites, present in certain foods (also used as food preservatives), seem to affect the incidence of stomach cancer. This may be because a number of genes are involved in determining the susceptibility of an individual to stomach cancer and also because interaction between genetic factors and dietary factors determine the time course and incidence of stomach cancer.

Association between stomach cancer and a few non-cancerous diseases has been observed. For example, the incidence of stomach cancer is higher in relatives of patients with pernicious anaemia (a serious form of anaemia) as well as achlorhydria (a pathological condition characterized by the absence of hydrochloric acid from the stomach) patients than in relatives of normal individuals, The incidence of stomach cancer seems to be higher in individuals of blood group A as compared to persons with other blood groups.

Colon Cancer

There is a strong hereditary predisposition towards polyposis of the colon, and pedigree analyses suggest an autosomal dominant mode of inheritance of this syndrome. Polyposis of the colon itself is a non-malignant tumour which appears by the time an individual reaches adulthood. One of the serious aspects of this syndrome is that it invariably leads to malignant adenocarcinoma of the colon by age 50. The population frequency of this disorder has been estimated to be about one per 10,000 births. The mutation rate of this dominant gene has been estimated to be within the range of 1×10^{-5} to 3×10^{-5} per gene per generation. Colon cancer is the second leading cause of cancer deaths in the USA (Figs. 6.1 and 6.2) and in the rest of the world.

Another genetic disease characterized by multiple polyps of the colon and occasionally of the small intestine is known as Gardner's syndrome (named after the discoverer). Here the gastrointestinal polyps occur in association with fibrosarcomas and osteomas of the facial bones. The onset of symptoms and age of diagnosis of Gardner's syndrome are rather similar to those in polyposis of the colon. Pedigree analyses indicate an autosomal dominant mode of inheritance for Gardner's syndrome.

In addition to the hereditary form, colon cancer may also arise spontaneously (non-hereditary form). In the hereditary form of colon cancer, the first mutation (dominant gene) is inherited via the germline (sex cells), while the second mutational event occurs in the somatic colonic cells, so that the end effect is that there are two copies of a defective gene. On the other hand, in the non-hereditary form of colon cancer, both mutational events would occur in the somatic cells of the colon. However, it is likely that the two mutational events may only produce polyps, and some additional genetic or developmental changes may be required to produce the malignant phenotype.

In breast cancer and stomach cancer (described in previous sections), a number of genes seem to determine susceptibility to these syndromes. Therefore, precise statements regarding their occurrence in a family are rather difficult to make. Nevertheless, relatives of probands from these two cancers are at a greater risk of developing the disease as compared to the general population. On the other hand, certain probability statements regarding the occurrence of colon cancer in a family can be made. Since polyposis of the colon is a dominantly inherited disorder, a cancer proband who marries a normal person will transmit the defective gene to 50 per cent of his or her children. On the other hand, when two individuals predisposed to cancer of the colon marry, they would transmit the defective genes to 75 per cent (assuming both parents are heterozygous) of their children; in other words, three-quarters of their children would be at a risk of developing colon cancer.

Recent molecular genetic studies have narrowed down the search for the defective gene involved in colon cancer. Current evidence suggests that the faulty gene predisposes individuals to colon cancer by actively promoting an accumulation of genetic errors in the genome, which, according to Bert Vogelstein of Johns Hopkins, Baltimore, eventually lead to malignant tumours of the colon.

Retinoblastoma

Retinoblastoma is a malignant tumour of the eye that usually occurs in children from the age of a few months to four years. It is an uncommon eye tumour that occurs at a frequency of 5 per 100,000 births, and accounts for 1 per cent of deaths from all cancer in early childhood and 5 per cent of all blindness in children. In the past this cancer was invariably fatal. However, with recent advances in early diagnosis and therapy, the number of survivors is increasing. Some of the survivors, who have married, have produced affected offspring.

At the familial level, retinoblastoma is an autosomal dominantly inherited disease, which means the defective gene is equally likely to be transmitted to male and female offspring through the germ cells. As it turns out, not all cases of retinoblastoma are hereditary. Sporadic (non-hereditary) cases of retinoblastoma also occur in the human population and these cases are usually unilateral, that is, affect only one eye. On the other hand, hereditary retinoblastoma is invariably bilateral, that is, both eyes are affected. In a number of cases of retinoblastoma, a specific chromosomal defect involving the deletion of the long arm of chromosome 13 has been observed. Further chromosomal characterization revealed that the deletion included a specific chromosome band 13q14, a genomic locus which determines one's susceptibility to retinoblastoma. By employing a closely linked gene for esterase D as a marker, certain molecular biologists have cloned the retinoblastoma gene from the 13q14 region.

However, the retinoblastoma gene is not an oncogene in itself. It is a tumour suppressor gene, which presumably regulates the expression of an oncogene located on another chromosome in the human genome. It has been postulated by Alfred Knudson that both hereditary and non-hereditary forms of retinoblastoma develop following loss or mutation of both copies of the retinoblastoma gene. In the hereditary form, the first mutation is inherited via germinal cells, while the second mutation occurs in the somatic retinal cells. On the other hand, in the non-hereditary form, both mutations occur in the somatic cells. It is interesting to note that retinoblastoma, which shows a dominant mode of inheritance at the familial level, actually results from recessive gene mutations at the cellular level, that is, loss or mutations of both copies of the retinoblastoma gene.

The transmission of the dominant gene in hereditary retinoblastoma follows the same pattern, as has been described for colon cancer, in families, that is, 50 per cent of the offspring are at risk of developing the disease when a carrier of the dominant gene marries a normal person. However, the sporadic or non-hereditary cases of retinoblastoma do not transmit the defective gene to the next generation, since, in these cases, the mutational events occur in the somatic cells which cannot be transmitted through the germ cells.

Xeroderma Pigmentosum

Xeroderma pigmentosum is a genetic disease which predisposes an individual to develop skin cancer following exposure to strong sunlight. This defect is found in one among approximately 250,000 individuals. Its occurrence is worldwide and in all races. Most patients having this genetic defect have an acute sensitivity to sunlight that is manifested in early life in the form of freckles which develop on the sun-exposed areas where the skin becomes dry and scaly. Later, skin cancer develops in the xeroderma pigmentosum patients. Studies on family history have indicated that xeroderma pigmentosum is inherited as a recessive trait.

Some insight has been gained into gene action in xeroderma pigmentosum. Normal persons have a mechanism for removal of DNA lesions caused by ultraviolet radiation. This removal is carried out by a multistep process called nucleotide excision repair (NER) and this process is regulated by excision repair genes. There are at least five steps involved in the NER process: (1) recognition of the lesion; (2) incision of the lesion; (3) excision of the lesion; (4) repair synthesis involving synthesis of DNA using undamaged complementary DNA template; and (5) ligation or joining of newly synthesized fragment(s) in place of discarded segments of DNA. The NER gene system is highly conserved in the mammals and has evolved as a mechanism for survival against genotoxic agents. However, mutations in the NER genes may lead to accumulation of lesions and errors in DNA, and, depending upon the severity of the defect, may be injurious to health or life-threatening. Xeroderma pigmentosum patients have a defect in the excision repair pathway for ultraviolet rays-induced damage to DNA, and therefore the faulty DNA is not repaired. The defect in DNA repair probably results in an increased mutation rate by ultraviolet light, and this leads to skin cancer in xeroderma pigmentosum patients.

Since xeroderma pigmentosum patients, who are homozygous (carry both the defective copies of the gene), seldom reproduce, they do not transmit the defective gene to the next generation. However, xeroderma pigmentosum trait carriers, who are heterozygous (carry one defective copy and a normal copy of the gene at a locus), may show freckling but do not necessarily develop skin cancer. These carriers can reproduce and when two carriers marry, they would transmit the defective copies of the gene to one quarter of their offspring. That is, one quarter of the children will be at risk of developing skin cancer. On the other hand, a marriage between a xeroderma pigmentosum carrier and a normal person would result in 50 per cent normal and 50 per cent xeroderma pigmentosum carrier children, who are not at risk of developing the xeroderma pigmentosum disease.

In xeroderma pigmentosum patients skin cancer is a preventable disease. Keeping away from sunlight or protection against sunlight (by wearing appropriate clothing) might reduce the risk of skin cancer in these patients.

GENETIC DEFECTS AND THE TIME COURSE OF HEREDITARY CANCER

It appears that in the hereditary cancers, in which specific tissues are tumour-prone, it is the proneness that seems to be the inherited component. However, for development of malignant tumours some additional genetic or developmental changes may be necessary. Therefore, it would appear that in the inherited cancers, one or more defective tissue-specific suppressor genes (regulatory genes) that are causally related to the disease are transmitted through the sex cells (germline) to the resulting zygote. After the initial determination in the embryo, the tumour-committed cells apparently undergo normal growth and development until a certain cell number or a certain stage of differentiation is attained either in the embryo, infant or adult individual before the appearance of tumours. In other words, in most instances, germline-conditioned cancers are programmed to develop in a specific tissue or organ, in a specific space, and at a specific time. Of these determinants, the first two, namely, specific tissue and specific space, are both determined at the time of fertilization; however, the time factor for the development of tumours may vary depending upon when the cells in the target tissue are subjected to physical, chemical, or biological agents. In highly malignant tumours, metastasis (migration of cancer cells from a cancerous tissue to other parts of the body through the blood stream) may occur. In that event, even the space no longer remains specific.

CHROMOSOME ABNORMALITIES AND CANCER

As already mentioned, chromosomes are the carriers of genetic information encoded in genes, which are located in a linear order on a chromosome. It is imperative for the normal functioning of the body that gene order, chromosome integrity, and chromosome balance be preserved. The normal chromosome number in the human body cells is 46. Changes in chromosome number or structure may have far-reaching consequences in genetic disease and behaviour. For example, Down's syndrome, characterized by mental retardation, growth failure, and slanting eyes, is associated with an extra chromosome 21, so that the patients with this syndrome have 47 instead of the normal 46 chromosomes. In an individual loss or addition of sex chromosomes (X or Y) has adverse effects on the sexual development and mental health. It has been observed that loss or deletion of a specific short segment of chromosome 5 in humans is associated with a syndrome known as *cri du chat* (cat cry). This syndrome is characterized by general retardation, low birth weight, a moon-like face, and the child's cry resembles that of a cat. Furthermore, on the basis of detailed observations made on human chromosomes and their abnormalities, it is apparent that almost every chromosome abnormality seems to be harmful for humans.

Chromosome abnormalities have also been frequently observed in human tumours. Earlier chromosome observations, based on conventional staining techniques, indicated that chromosome variability results from random events occurring during the progression (malignant transformation) of most tumours. However, following the advent of newer staining procedures of chromosome analysis, it was found that specific types of chromosome abnormalities, a number of them associated with fragile sites, were subsequently found to occur frequently in a number of human cancers. Now, with the new procedures, it is possible to identify not only individual chromosomes but also small segments (single bands) of each human chromosome -- something not possible with conventional staining techniques -- whereby an entire chromosome is stained uniformly and the fine details are not discernible. By employing high-resolution banding techniques, it has been possible to show that certain specific chromosome abnormalities occur frequently in certain human cancers. From this category of cancers, chronic myelogenous leukaemia, Burkitt's lymphoma, and meningiomas will now be discussed.

Chronic Myelogenous Leukaemia

Chronic myelogenous leukaemia (CML) is a disease resulting due to abnormally proliferating white blood cells. About 90 per cent of the patients with CML have a so-called 'Philadelphia chromosome' (discovered in Philadelphia) resulting from translocation between chromosomes 9 and 22 (9;22) (q34;q11). This translocation involves the transfer of q34, carrying the proto-oncogene *c-abl* locus, to the breakpoint cluster region (bcr) located in band q11 of the chromosome 22 (Fig. 6.4). This chromosome abnormality is only found in the white blood cells, and not in any other tissue of the body. It is interesting to note that, in most cases, both the twins of a monozygotic pair develop CML. However, several cases have been reported where only one of the twins is afflicted, and only the CML-affected twin possesses the Philadelphia chromosome. Such observations on the presence of the chromosome abnormality in the proliferating white blood cells and the data on twins tend to support the notion that CML arises post-zygotically (i.e., after birth) in individuals and, therefore, is a non-hereditary genetic disease.

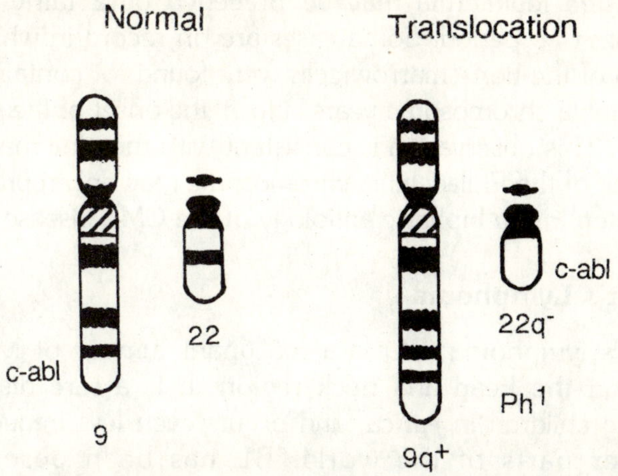

Fig. 6.4 Diagrammatic representation of a translocation between human chromosomes 9 and 22 in the chronic myelogenous leukaemia (CML). The translocation involves the transfer of tip of chromosome 9 ($9q^+$) and a large part of chromosome 22 ($22q^-$), resulting in a relatively small chromosome 22 known as the Philadelphia (Ph^1) chromosome. The Ph^1 chromosome is present in more than 90 per cent of the patients with CML.

Further, it has been observed that transformation from the chronic phase to the acute phase ('blastic crisis') of the CML disease seems to be accompanied by the presence of extra chromosomes 8, 17, 19 and 22. Acute leukaemia strikes only when these additional chromosome abnormalities have occurred in cells having the Philadelphia chromosome. This suggests that transition from normal to acute leukaemia might involve at least two major phases: the first is involved in the 'initiation' and the second in the 'development' of the CML disease. Genetic changes in the chronic phase involving chromosomes 9;22 may constitute the initiation phase, while those changes occurring during the blastic crisis may represent the developmental phase. There are indications that clinically manifested leukaemia may be preceded by a fairly long symptom-free period. Some cases are on record in which a portion of the bone marrow cells were found to contain the Philadelphia chromosome years before the onset of the CML disease. This observation is consistent with the idea that the presence of the Philadelphia chromosome may only represent a first step in the biphasic aetiology of the CML disease.

Burkitt's Lymphoma

Burkitt's lymphoma (BL) is a malignant tumour of lymph glands in the head and neck region. It is a rare disease afflicting children in Africa, and occurs even less frequently in other parts of the world. BL has been observed predominantly in children between the ages of 2 and 12, with a peak incidence at 7 years. Adults may also be occasionally affected by this cancer. In BL virtually 100 per cent of the patients carry a specific chromosome abnormality. About 80 per cent of BL patients exhibit a translocation of a specific chromosome band (q24) from chromosome 8 to the distal region (q32) of chromosome 14. This translocation, according to recent experimental evidence, involves the transfer of a proto-oncogene *c-myc* located in band q24 on chromosome 8 to distal band q32 of chromosome 14 (8q24;14q32). The remaining 20 per cent of the BL patients also exhibit translocations between 8 and 22 (8q24;22q11) and 2 and 8 (2q11;8q24). Thus, in the majority of cases, the proto-oncogene *c-myc* from chromosome 8 is either translocated to another location, or another chromosomal band translocated to the *c-myc* locus. The only other chromosome abnormality observed with a noticeable frequency involves an extra chromosome 7. These observations suggest that the translocation involving the *c-myc* locus may initiate the oncogenesis process and some further genetic changes may be necessary for malignant transformation.

Meningioma

Meningioma (MG) is a benign tumour of the brain. It arises in the meningeal covering of the brain. In most cases of MG, the primary change most frequently involves one chromosome, i.e., chromosome 22: one entire chromosome is missing or the distal segment of chromosome 22 is lost. In contrast to the findings in CML (with the Philadelphia chromosome), however, in MG the deleted segment of chromosome 22 does not appear to be transferred to any other chromosome in the human complement. Besides the primary genetic change that involves the loss of chromosome 22, or part thereof, there are additional chromosome changes that occur, the most common one being the loss of chromosomes 1, 8, and 9. Since a majority of tumour cells analysed from MG patients reveal a stemline (all cells arise from a common stem cell; clonal origin) distribution in the 45 chromosome range, it appears that the secondary changes involving losses of chromosomes 1, 8, and 9 may occur individually in separate cells and perhaps not altogether in the cells of the same tumour.

More recently a dominant gene, NF2, has been located on chromosome 22 which is involved in neurofibromatosis 2, characterized by a predisposition to tumours of the nervous system, including meningiomas. Thus, gross deletions involving the entire chromosome 22 or the region carrying the NF2 gene seem to be the critical somatic mutation in meningiomas.

CHROMOSOME ABERRATIONS MAY CAUSE IMPAIRMENT OF SUPPRESSOR GENES

When we consider the non-random nature of chromosome abnormalities in certain human cancers, such as chronic myelogenous leukaemia, Burkitt's lymphoma, and meningiomas, it is relevant to ask: Are these specific chromosome aberrations the cause or result of neoplastic development? Chronic myelogenous leukaemia, Burkitt's lymphoma, as well as many other human cancers, are clonal in origin, that is, they are derived from single cells, and therefore, might originate as a result of mutational events. Since specific chromosome abnormalities (mutations), involving certain proto-oncogenes, are present in primary tumours, it might be argued that these are somehow causally involved in the origin of cancer; that specific primary chromosome changes may be relevant to the initiation phase of certain sporadic human cancers. Thus, it would appear that the specific chromosomes involved in these cancers probably carry the genes necessary for the prevention of tumour formation, and loss or mutation of these suppressor genes may lead to the onset of tissue-specific malignancies.

7

Environmental Factors and Cancer (I)

OCCUPATIONS, CUSTOMS AND HABITS

A large number of agents present in our environment have been implicated in the causation of human cancer. Epidemiological data suggests that 70 to 90 per cent of the human cancers are due to carcinogens in the environment, and, therefore, in principle, these cancers are preventable. This has given rise to worldwide concern about environmental pollutants and their hazardous effect on humans. While earlier clinical observations were mostly derived from those human cancers that were occupational in origin, later investigations were extended to ascertain the relationship between cancer and man's general, that is, non-occupational, environment. Included in the non-occupational category are the cancers associated with customs, habits, drugs, pollutants in the environment, such as pesticides, detergents, fumes from factories and automobiles, industrial wastes and byproducts, contaminants, food additives, and therapeutic agents. We can be sure that the list of pollutants will continue to grow in the future with more industrialization and greater production and utilization of atomic energy, unless we make serious efforts to keep our environment (air, water and soil) relatively clean. Unfortunately, some of the new synthetic chemicals and their degradation products in our environment may not only be carcinogenic, but also toxic. Human beings have traversed a very long path starting from the remote past of their primitive ancestors to almost the twenty-first century. To make their living conditions congenial and comfortable, humans have made tremendous progress in science and technology. But, as one knows, everything has a price! Obviously, with greater advances in science and technology there will be problems peculiar to new kinds of environmental pollutants. Thus, it is extremely difficult to envisage a pollution-free environment. Therefore, our goal should be to minimize the extent of environmental pollution and thus keep a check on the diseases related to such pollution.

It should be pointed out that in human cancers associated with the occupational and non-occupational environments, the environmental agents are *suspected* to be the causative agents. However, in most cases, these agents have been tested and confirmed for their carcinogenic properties in experimental model systems. Due to ethical reasons, since human beings cannot be used for testing environmental carcinogenesis, the experimental research in this area is restricted to animals, such as mice, rats, hamsters, fishes and monkeys. The knowledge gained from such experimental studies in animals not only would be of immense value for an understanding of the mode of action of the environmental agent in transformation of a normal cell into a cancer cell, but would also be valuable for designing approaches for the prevention and control of human cancer.

OCCUPATIONAL CANCERS

Occupational cancers are those cancers which are related to the professional activity of individuals whether in industry or in scientific research. During the occupational period the individuals are constantly exposed to a carcinogenic agent and generally develop cancer many years after their first contact with the agent. Clinicians and epidemiologists became aware of occupational cancers when many individuals working in the same industry were reported to have developed a particular type of cancer. The number of cases were far too large to attribute to chance alone. A cause-and-effect relationship between a carcinogenic agent and a particular type of cancer seemed more probable. In principle, therefore, occupational cancers are preventable once the risk of a carcinogenic agent has been evaluated.

Scrotal cancer is a good example of the relationship between an occupation and the disease. More than 200 years ago a British clinician named Percival Pott published the first carefully documented report on the association between an environmental agent and human cancer. He reported that chimney-sweeps were prone to develop skin cancer of the scrotum. During that period it was a common practice in England to lower very small boys down the chimneys to clean them. Prolonged exposure of the chimney-sweeps to soot from the chimneys of open fireplaces resulted in a high incidence of skin cancer of the scrotum decades after the first exposure to soot. Subsequently, a wide range of occupational cancers have since been identified and investigated.

People *have* to work for their livelihood and are often unaware of the consequences of the long-term contact and exposure to certain chemicals that may be directly or indirectly related to their occupations. One such consequence is *skin cancer* which has been found frequently in workers in the coal tar and creosote industry, and seems to be associated with skin exposure to polycyclic hydrocarbons in the tar and soot. Another occupational cancer is *urinary bladder cancer* which develops more frequently in people working in the dyestuff and rubber industries. This type of cancer is apparently related to the exposure to amines. It has been observed that in comparison to the general public, people who have inhaled dust from chromate ore or those who work in the asbestos industry are more prone to develop *lung cancer*.

We, as consumers, cannot imagine a world devoid of plastic products. Plastic industries have been set up in almost all the countries of the world, and the existence of many people depends on them. It is a paradox that an industry which provides for their livelihood may also be the cause of their suffering and death. It has been observed that workers involved in the manufacture of polyvinyl chloride, a gaseous chemical used in the plastic industry, are at a greater risk of contracting *liver cancer*. Another type of cancer common among workers in the nickel ore plants is the *cancer of the nasal sinuses*. This form of cancer is also prevalent in the hardwood furniture and leather goods industries. This is due to the exposure to agents in the isopropyl oil used in these industries. It is tragic that during the earlier part of the twentieth century, workers in the watch-making industry who ingested radioactive substances while painting luminous dials of watches with a dilute radium solution became victims of *bone cancer*. All these examples underline the hazards that accompany an occupation. Therefore, to safeguard the lives of numerous workers involved in these and similar occupations, it is of utmost importance that adequate safety means be provided and more research carried out for environmental-friendly and safer industries. After all, as mentioned earlier, occupational cancers are, by and large, preventable.

CANCERS ASSOCIATED WITH CUSTOMS AND HABITS

Cancers in this category are associated with customs and habits which are peculiar to different geographical regions of the world. That is not to say that the cancers described in this category do not occur in other parts of the world, but rather that the incidence of such cancers is comparatively higher in certain regions due to the constant exposure of the individuals to certain environmental agents. In other words, there is a striking difference in the geographical distribution of various forms of cancer; this is an observation consistent with the notion that environmental factors are involved in the aetiology of human cancer. Some of the cancers associated with customs and habits are described as follows.

'Kanghri-burn' cancer is prevalent in north-west India especially Kashmir. In order to keep themselves warm during the freezing cold months of winter, the natives of this region bind small earthen ovens (*kanghri*) containing burning charcoal around their waists. The *kanghri*-burn cancer commonly develops in the skin of the abdomen in contact with the hot earthen oven years after the first exposure.

The *betel quid cancer* or cancer of the mouth is common among the betel quid chewers in India, especially those in Travancore (Kerala). It has been estimated that about 75 per cent of the cancers of the buccal cavity in the mouth diagnosed in Travancore have been attributed to persistent chewing of 'pan' containing betel nuts, cheap tobacco, and lime from the crushed shells. Although the cancer of the mouth from Travancore is commonly known as the 'betel quid' cancer, the carcinogenic action may be attributed to the tobacco in the quid.

The cancer of the palate is common in certain areas of South Asia. An unusual and curious custom locally known as *chutta* is practised by certain native groups in South Asia. It involves smoking cigars with the burning end held in the mouth. This practice has resulted in a high incidence of cancer of the palate known as '*reverse smoking*' cancer.

Skin cancer is particularly common in sailors due to excessive exposure to strong sunlight. Skin cancer is also prevalent in Australia and other countries with sunny climates. This type of cancer is largely confined to individuals with light skin and is rather less frequent in dark-skinned people. The carcinogenic action is attributed to the ultraviolet radiation in the sunlight.

Cancer of the penis is common in uncircumcized individuals, who do not practise adequate personal hygiene. Cancer of the penis is rather rare among Jews, and less common in Moslems. It is a custom among Jews to circumcize a male child one week after birth, and the Moslems also follow the same custom of circumcision later in childhood. Apparently circumcision keeps the penis relatively clean and minimizes the risk of penis cancer.

Individuals who smoke tobacco are at a greater risk of developing *lung cancer*. The incidence of lung cancer varies in different countries. However, the higher incidence of lung cancer has been positively correlated to heavy tobacco smoking. Tobacco smoking causes lung cancer in both males and females (see Chapter 8 for more details).

8

Environmental Factors and Cancer (II)

TOBACCO, DIET, AND OTHER POTENTIALLY CARCINOGENIC SUBSTANCES

Science and technology have played an important role in changing human lifestyles. Rapid transportation systems have dramatically altered human diet, since all kinds of exotic foods are now easily available. In order to lengthen the storage life of exotic, and also non-exotic foods, they are treated with chemicals or radiation. Animals are regularly fed with chemicals/drugs to increase their body fat, milk supply and to make them resistant to diseases. Crops are sprayed with pesticides to protect them from insects and other diseases to increase their yield, and thereby feed the teeming millions. Socio-economic reasons have already forced most family members to take up jobs, and as a result, people have less and less time to cook food. Readily prepared meals, canned food, frozen foods, etc., are available in the supermarkets in the industrialized countries, and their shelf-life has to be maintained by adding chemical preservatives. If we take time off and seriously consider all the things we consume in the forms of foods, drinks, smoke and drugs (medicinal), we will be surprised at the large amounts of chemicals we bombard our body cells with. Of course, as we enter the next century, our diet will change considerably firstly due to the population explosion and secondly maybe because of expansion in space travel. Well, for the time being, let us take into account the three major environmental factors, namely, tobacco, diet and drugs, that seem to influence the development of cancer. The subject of tobacco-related cancer has been extensively investigated during the past 40 years. The evidence for the diet- and drug-associated cancers has also been forthcoming in recent years.

TOBACCO

Cigarette Smoking

It has been known for over 100 years that persistent chewing of 'pan' (betel nut quid) in certain parts of Asia, particularly India, was associated with cancer of the mouth. It was suspected that crude tobacco included in the 'pan' was the major culprit causing mouth cancer. The tobacco-cancer connection was largely neglected until a rapid and increased incidence of lung cancer deaths occurred during the present century, and it was noted that a great majority of the lung cancer patients were cigarette smokers. Cigarette smoking in men began around the time of World War I, while this practice became fashionable with women just prior to World War II. The trend in smoking and the incidence of lung cancer have both increased linearly and proportionately in the last several decades, and lung cancer now accounts for one-third of all cancer deaths in the USA, and about half of all cancer deaths in England. The incidence of lung cancer is relatively higher in men as compared to women. This is due to the fact that women started the cigarette-smoking habit much later than men, and probably do not smoke as much as men do. Lung cancer, of course, does not develop in a week or a month after one begins the smoking habit, but rather years (10-15) after one has first started smoking, since this cancer develops after a long 'latent period'. The risk of dying from lung cancer increases 10-fold to 50-fold depending upon the smoking habit (i.e., number of cigarettes smoked per day) and the environment one lives in. In addition to tobacco smoke, urban air pollution (exhausts from industry and automobiles) may also be contributing to the increased incidence of lung cancer. It is also known that exposure to asbestos and cigarette smoking together produces a synergistic effect in the causation of lung cancer. Asbestos workers who smoke have an eight-fold increased risk of dying from lung cancer as compared to cigarette smokers who do not work with asbestos, and these workers are at about 90 times the risk compared to those who neither smoke nor are exposed to asbestos.

Tobacco smoking is a highly addictive habit. Humans are victims of their habits, and it is very difficult to give up addictive habits in the absence of acceptable substitutes. The production of low-tar cigarettes was intended to offer a reasonable substitute, but the new type of cigarettes also posed certain risks to health. Current data indicate that a heavy smoker who stops smoking will decrease his lung cancer risk considerably. The quantity of tobacco smoked in the rich countries has been decreasing over the past few decades. However, in the Third World countries, tobacco consumption has been increasing. Tobacco smoking is not only hazardous to those who smoke, but is also harmful for non-smokers or passive smokers who inhale the smoke. Besides, being a high risk factor for lung cancer, tobacco smoke also seems to be associated with cancers of the oral cavity, oesophagus, pancreas, kidney, and urinary bladder, as well as emphysema and coronary heart disease.

Pipe and Cigar Smoking

The incidence of lung cancer in individuals with a history of pipe or cigar smoking is significantly higher than that of individuals who have never smoked. However, the pipe and cigar smokers are at a relatively lower risk of contracting lung cancer compared to cigarette smokers. As it turns out, most pipe or cigar smokers may or may not inhale the smoke, while most cigarette smokers do inhale it. Therefore, those pipe or cigar smokers who do inhale the smoke are at as great a risk of developing lung cancer as cigarette smokers.

DIET

Diet has been implicated in the aetiology of a number of human cancers. Several lines of evidence suggest that cancers of the stomach, the colon, and the liver are associated with certain dietary components. In addition, cancers of the breast, prostate, and ovary have also been linked to dietary factors. The poor and the rich of this world are at high risks for different cancers listed earlier, and the difference in incidence, in part, may be determined by the nutritional economies. For example, cancers of the stomach and liver are the diseases of the lower socio-economic groups. Cancer of the stomach is prevalent in Japan, the western part of South America, part of Central America, and northern and eastern Europe. Cancer of the liver is common in parts of East Africa and South-East Asia. On the other hand, cancers of the colon, breast, prostate, pancreas and ovary are the diseases of affluent societies and are common in the USA, western Europe, Australia, New Zealand and Argentina. These geographical distributions of cancer have been shown to be influenced by environmental factors, particularly dietary variables.

Aflatoxin

A naturally occurring carcinogenic agent that is widespread as a food contaminant is *aflatoxin*, a metabolic product of the fungus *Aspergillus flavus*. The carcinogenic potential of aflatoxin (B1) was discovered under somewhat unusual circumstances. In 1960 two serious epidemics occurred, one resulting in the death of some 100,000 turkeys and ducks in the British farms and the second in a loss of 50 to 75 per cent of rainbow trout in the American hatcheries. The cause of the epidemic in both cases was subsequently traced to the contamination of the animal diet (peanut meal for the farm birds and the cottonseed meal for the fish) by aflatoxin, which produced liver necrosis and liver cancer. It is now known that minute doses of aflatoxin can cause cancer of the liver in a variety of animals.

The fungus *Aspergillus flavus* does not normally attack the living plants, but is a frequent contaminant of the food grains (groundnut, cotton seed, corn, soyabean, etc.) stored under high humid and high temperature conditions. Therefore, aflatoxin-contaminated foodstuff might constitute a major cause of liver cancer in humans. Human liver cells contain the enzyme necessary for conversion of aflatoxin to its active carcinogenic form (epoxy derivatives). A higher incidence of liver cancer in the inhabitants of South-East Asia (Thailand), and Africa (Kenya, Swaziland, and Mozambique) seems to be directly related to the amount of aflatoxin in the diet. Therefore, contamination of stored food grains and staple foods under the hot and humid conditions of the tropics by aflatoxin (and other fungal products) poses a serious health hazard for humans and farm animals.

Meat and Animal Fat

It has been suggested that there is a relationship between dietary components and certain types of cancer, particularly the cancers of the colon, rectum, stomach, pancreas, prostate, ovary, and breast. The incidence of colon cancer among women from different geographical regions of the world seems to be closely correlated to per capita meat consumption in those countries (Fig. 8.1). The women from countries with a higher per capita meat consumption of 200 to 300 grams per day as in Canada, the USA, and New Zealand have a considerably higher incidence of colon cancer as compared to those from countries with rather low per capita meat consumption of 20 to 100 grams per day, as in Nigeria, Japan, Colombia, Chile and Finland. The relationship of colon cancer and high meat intake is clearly evident when one compares New Zealand and Nigeria. It is interesting to observe that the cancer of the colon is almost 40-fold higher in the women from New Zealand with the highest per capita meat consumption (about 300 grams per day) as compared to the women from Nigeria with the lowest per capita meat consumption (about 20 grams per day). Since high meat consumption and low cereal intake may often go together, the cancer of the colon might also be attributed to a low cereal diet. In general, the incidence and risk of cancer of the colon or large intestine seem to be higher in the industrialized countries where the diet consists of meat and processed and canned foods, but is relatively low in cereals and indigestible fibre. On the other hand, the incidence and risk of colon cancer are relatively low in populations whose diet consists of natural unprocessed foods and cereals with adequate amounts of indigestible fibre, but, at the same time, the diet is also low in meat intake.

A high intake of dietary meat, animal fat, particularly from beef, and possibly dietary fibre deficiency are strongly associated with cancer of the colon. Evidence tends to favour dietary fat, particularly that derived from beef, as the major ingredient in the causation of colon cancer. Fats by themselves are not carcinogenic, but may affect the cholesterol and bile salt metabolism and the decomposition of bacterial flora of the colon, which, in turn, may metabolize the precarcinogens

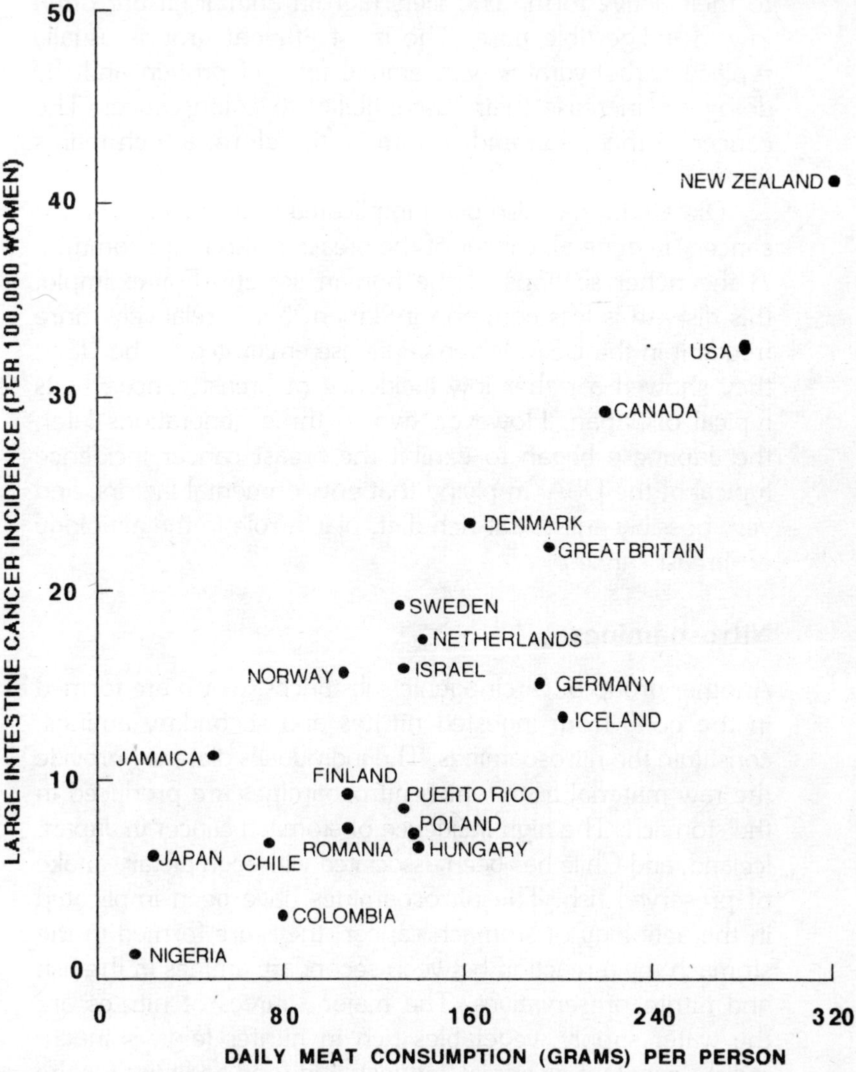

Fig. 8.1 Relationship between daily meat consumption and incidence of cancer of the large intestine in women from 21 nations. Higher meat consumption seems to increase the risk of large intestine cancer (modified from Armstrong and Doll, *Int. J. Cancer,* 1975).

to their active form. The diets high in animal fat are often low in indigestible fibre. The most affluent groups usually replace carbohydrates with animal fat and protein and, by doing so, increase their susceptibility to colon cancer. The cancer of the colon and rectum is, therefore, a 'rich man's disease'.

Dietary fat has also been implicated in the case of breast cancer. In general, cancer of the breast is also more common in the richer sections of the human society. For example, this disease is less common in Japan, but is relatively more frequent in the USA. When Japanese emigrated to the USA, they showed a rather low incidence of breast cancer, as is typical of Japan. However, two to three generations later, the Japanese began to exhibit the breast cancer incidence typical of the USA, implying that environmental factors, and very possibly animal fat-rich diet, play a role in the aetiology of breast cancer.

Nitrosoamines

Another group of carcinogenic substances, which are formed in the body from ingested nitrites and secondary amines, constitute the nitrosoamines. The individual's diet may provide the raw material from which nitrosoamines are produced in the stomach. The high incidence of stomach cancer in Japan, Iceland, and Chile has been associated with high dietary intake of preserved fish. The nitrosoamines have been implicated in the aetiology of stomach cancer; they are formed in the stomach by a reaction between secondary amines in the fish and nitrite preservatives. The major sources of nitrites are the water supply, vegetables rich in nitrites (e.g., spinach, radish, eggplant or brinjal, lettuce), and food additives for the preservation of fish, meat, etc. Nitrites can also be formed from nitrates in the mouth as a result of bacterial metabolism. The main source of secondary amines are fish, cereals, tea, tobacco, etc., and in the form of certain pharmaceutical drugs (for example, Piperazine, used against worms in the stomach).

Cooking meat and fish also provides a source of secondary amines. The nitrosoamines are a group of powerful chemicals and produce cancer in a variety of organs in many animal species. Therefore, nitrosoamines may also cause cancer in humans.

That diet plays an important role in the aetiology of stomach cancer is evident by the decreasing trends in the stomach cancer in certain countries. Stomach cancer is common in relatively poor populations of Japan and northern Europe. However, it has become progressively less common in western Europe and the USA, and even among the Japanese immigrants in the USA. This disease seems to occur in those Japanese who tend to eat pickled vegetables and dried and salted fish. But the incidence of stomach cancer is low in those who eat a more balanced Western diet consisting of tomatoes, corn, celery, onion, and lettuce. The reduction in stomach cancer in the USA and western Europe may in part be due to small amounts of Vitamin C present in the fresh vegetables, which may inhibit the formation of nitrosoamines in the stomach. The reduction in the incidence of stomach cancer may also be attributed to better processing and preservation of food material.

Other Dietary Factors

Relationships between other dietary factors and several human cancers have also been suggested. For example, consumption of beverages has been associated with the cancer of the oral cavity, oesophagus and liver. Charcoal broiling of meat and fish leads to production of highly mutagenic pyrolytic products in the broiled foods, and these products may cause cancer of the gastrointestinal tract. Caffeine, one of the major constituents of coffee, has been shown to be mutagenic and carcinogenic in animal tests, and drinking excessive coffee may be potentially hazardous (carcinogenic) for humans. Production of caffeine-free coffee may be a reasonable substitute in this direction. Even the water we drink may not be clean. Most rivers in the industrialized cities are heavily polluted with industrial and municipal wastes. Even chlorination of drinking water, particularly if the source is heavily polluted with organic chemicals, results in the production of chlorinated hydrocarbons, some of which may be carcinogenic.

POTENTIALLY CARCINOGENIC SUBSTANCES FOR HUMANS

There are a number of substances used in food preservatives, pesticides, detergents, and therapeutic drugs, which may be 'potentially carcinogenic' for humans, since they are known to be carcinogenic in the case of laboratory animals. Whether or not they are actually carcinogenic in humans needs to be pursued in order to establish some cause-and-effect relationship for specific cancers. The category 'potentially carcinogenic' would also include many of the naturally occurring substances in the human environment. However, the use of the term 'potentially carcinogenic' is commonly restricted to synthetic products introduced in our environment such as: (1) food additives to improve the storage properties, flavour, texture, and colour of the foods; (2) pesticides, detergents; and (3) drugs for medicinal purposes.

Routine carcinogenicity testing of 'potentially carcinogenic' substances is generally regulated by the governmental agencies (for example, the Food and Drug Administration in the USA). Hundreds of chemicals are now being tested at many laboratories in the USA under the sponsorship of the National Institute of Health (NIH) carcinogenic programme. The purpose of such carcinogenic tests, which are rigorous, expensive and often time-consuming, is to determine whether a certain product is 'safe' for human use. The term 'safe' in the present context could only imply that a certain product is relatively harmless and may not pose health hazards. In the USA, the Delaney Amendment to the Federal Food, Drugs and Cosmetic Act expressly prohibits the use of food additives that have been known to be carcinogenic to humans or to experimental animals. The World Health Organization has established the International Agency for Research on Cancer (IARC) in Lyon, France, with the explicit objective of encouraging international collaboration on cancer epidemiology, and carcinogenic testing, in the human beings' environment.

Food Additives

Perhaps 'butter yellow' (4-dimethyaminoazobenzene), which was used to give a richer colour to butter and margarine, was the first 'potentially carcinogenic' substance for humans, as determined by animal tests. 'Butter yellow' is a potent liver carcinogen for the laboratory animals when administered at a high dose level. Although the amounts of the 'butter yellow' added to butter or margarine were very small, its use has since been discontinued.

The synthetic colouring agents used in items such as confectionery, beverages, canned fruits and vegetables have also been suspected to be possible carcinogens. One such synthetic agent (auramine) has been shown to cause cancer of the liver and lymphoid tissue in mice. Another colouring agent, FD & C Violet No. 1, long used as the stamping dye for meat inspection, was withdrawn in the USA on the basis of preliminary carcinogenic tests on animals. In addition, certain sweetening agents added to the food, such as dulcin which causes liver cancer and cyclamate which induces bladder cancer in animals, have long been banned in many countries.

Other potentially carcinogenic food additives include: (a) thickening agents (such as carboxyethylcellulose) used in icecream, which induces cancer at the site of injection in laboratory animals; (b) an emulsifying agent (Tween 60), which acts as a promoter of skin cancer; (c) a preservative (hexamethyenetramine) for fish, meat, and pickles, which produces sarcomas in rats at the site of injection; and (d) a synthetic estrogen (diethylstilbestrol) used for caponizing poultry (some of which may be accidentally consumed by humans) has been shown to cause cancer of the breast and other organs in mice.

Food Contaminants: Pesticides

The pesticides which indirectly become a part of our diet concern humans not only as potential carcinogens, but also as toxic compounds. Some of the pesticides, such as DDT, tend to accumulate in the environment, since they are not degraded by bacteria in the soil or water, or by animal or plant metabolism. DDT is a widely used insecticide, which produces liver cancer and lung cancer in laboratory animals. Another insecticide, aldrin, produces liver cancer in mice even at very low concentrations. Aramite, used against mites, produces cancer of the liver and other organs in rats and dogs, while thiourea, used as a fungicide in the case of citrus fruits, produces cancer of the liver and thyroid in rats. It is interesting to note that liver seems to be the main target for the carcinogen action of most pesticides, primarily because most foreign chemicals tend to accumulate in this organ.

Medicinal Agents

There are a large number of agents used in medicinal drugs and for diagnostic procedures which pose potential carcinogenic hazards for humans. During the last three to four decades X-rays were used for diagnostic purposes in pregnant women in western Europe and North America. This practice of exposing expecting mothers to X-rays probably resulted in an increased incidence of cancer, particularly leukaemia, in their children. X-rays are powerful carcinogenic agents and, therefore, should be employed for diagnostic purposes only when their use is *fully justifiable*. Ultrasonic waves have now largely replaced X-rays as diagnostic agents in pregnant women.

There are a number of therapeutic agents which carry a carcinogenic risk for humans, most of which produce tumours in test animals. These agents include: (1) Fowler's solution (containing arsenic), used for treating skin problems, may cause skin cancer; (2) azathioprine, an immunosuppressive drug, may cause lymphomas; (3) chloramphenicol, an antibiotic, may cause leukaemia; (4) estrogen (diethylstilbestrol), administered to pregnant women for averting threatened abortion, may cause vaginal carcinoma during the gestation period years later in a small proportion of the daughters treated with the estrogen; and (4) thorotrast, used as a 'contrast' medium in diagnostic radiology, may cause liver cancer in humans. A more detailed list of chemical carcinogens suspected of causing cancer in humans is provided in Table 8.1.

Table 8.1 Chemical agents that exhibit carcinogenic risk for humans associated with occupation, lifestyle, pesticides, and therapeutic agents (*source*: R. Doll, *Nature*, 1977; H. Pitot, In: *Cancer – Principles and Practices of Oncology*, edited by De Vita *et al.*, 2nd edition, 1989; modified).

Chemical	*Site of cancer*
Occupational	
Polycyclic hydrocarbons	Skin
Benzidine	Urinary bladder
Soot, tar	Skin
Chromate ore	Lung
Asbestos	Lung

(cont'd)

Chemical	Site of cancer
Nickel ore	Nasal sinuses, lung
Vinyl chloride	Liver
Aromatic amines	Bladder
Lifestyle and Diet	
Aflatoxin	Liver
'Pan' (betel nut quid)	Mouth
Nitrosoamines	Stomach, liver, kidney
Tobacco smoking	Lung, mouth, oesophagus
Alcoholic beverages	Oesophagus, liver
Dietary fat	Colon, rectum, breast
Cyclamate	Urinary bladder
Pesticides	
DDT	Liver
Aldrin	Liver
Aramite	Liver
Therapeutic (medicinal)	
Fowler's solution (arsenic)	Skin
Coal tar ointment	Skin
Estrogen	Breast
Diethylstilbestrol (synthetic estrogen)	Vagina
Immunosuppressive drugs (Azathioprine)	Lymphomas

(cont'd)

Chemical	*Site of cancer*
Phenacetin	Kidney
Thorotrast	Liver
Chloramphenicol	Leukaemia
Chlornaphazine	Bladder
Alkylating agents (cyclophosphamide, melphalan)	Bladder
Oxymetholone	Liver

9

Environmental Factors and Cancer (III)

CHEMICAL CARCINOGENS

A number of chemicals pose carcinogenic risks for humans. Some of these chemicals occur naturally in our environment, while others are man-made. Most of the carcinogenic chemicals must be converted into their ultimate reactive form in the host before they can transform normal cells into cancer cells. By contrast, a small proportion of chemicals are direct-acting carcinogens which do not require the participation of the host organism to produce their ultimate active form. In this case, the chemical itself is the ultimate carcinogen and directly acts on the cell targets to convert the normal cell into a cancer cell. Some carcinogenic chemicals are active in producing cancer only in certain specific tissues or organs, while others may induce cancer in a variety of different tissues or organs. Carcinogenic chemicals range from inorganic substances, such as arsenic and asbestos, to organic substances which may be structurally simple, as urethane, to structurally complex [such as benz(a)pyrene].

Ever since the discovery by Percival Pott in 1775 that the incidence of scrotal cancer in British chimney-sweeps could be attributed to constant exposure to coal tar in the soot, a large number of compounds of proven carcinogenicity in humans (see Table 8.1), together with others with a lesser degree of certainty, have emerged, and this list continues to grow. So far more than 1000 chemicals have been shown to be carcinogenic in animal tests, of which a considerable number exist in the human environment.

CONVERSION OF CHEMICAL CARCINOGENS INTO AN ACTIVE FORM

There is absolutely nothing in the structure of highly diverse carcinogenic chemicals which is common to all of them. However, it now appears that the great majority, and perhaps all, of the carcinogenic chemicals are similar to one another in that they contain electron-deficient atoms (electrophiles) in their molecules, which then attack the electron-rich atoms (nucleophiles) found in the macromolecules (DNA, RNA, and proteins) of a cell. Of these macromolecules, DNA seems to be the main target of chemical carcinogens. The direct-working chemical carcinogens are already in the electrophilic state when they enter a cell, while many others require structural modifications before conversion into the carcinogenic or electrophilic form. Therefore, transformation of a normal cell into a cancer cell, in most cases, depends upon the presence or inducibility of appropriate enzymes required to convert a chemical into its carcinogenic form. The most important of these are a set of oxidizing enzymes known collectively as 'microsomal mixed-function oxygenases' which are present in moderate amounts in the liver and kidney, where foreign chemicals mainly accumulate, and in lower concentrations in most other cell types. Microsomes are subcellular particles that act as the seat of protein synthesis.

It is indeed ironical that the enzymes that activate many chemicals to their carcinogenic form are those whose primary function is the detoxification and disposal of foreign chemicals. Disposal of chemicals is accomplished by oxidation of functional groups of foreign molecules, which convert the foreign chemicals to more polar compounds. These compounds get attached to sugars or other molecules, which render them soluble so that they can be secreted.

Conversion of a Pesticide

One of the best examples of the activity of microsomal oxygenases involves the conversion of 2-acetylaminofluorene (AAF) to its active form. This compound was originally intended as a pesticide for domestic use, but, fortunately, animal tests for carcinogenicity were carried out in time, and thus it was never marketed. In spite of its low toxicity, AAF was found to be a potent chemical carcinogen and produced tumours in a great majority of organs, including the liver, the urinary bladder, the mammary gland, the intestine, and the brain, in a large variety of animals such as mouse, rat, hamster, rabbit, fowl, cat, and dog.

Conversion of Tobacco Smoke

Another good example is the metabolism of benz(a)pyrene, one of the major carcinogens produced due to incomplete combustion of tobacco smoke. Benz(a)pyrene is converted into its active form by a group of microsomal oxygenases called aryl hydrocarbon hydralases (AHH), and, in humans, a single genetic locus or a relatively few genes determine the level of inducibility of AHH. It has been suggested by G. Kellermann *et al*. that those individuals who have inherited the gene(s) for synthesizing relatively high amounts of inducible AHH activity are at a greater risk of developing lung cancer. On the other hand, individuals who carry the genetic information for a relatively low inducibility of AHH seem to be much less susceptible to the carcinogenic effect of the cigarette smoke.

SCREENING OF CHEMICALS FOR CARCINOGENICITY

The screening of chemicals for carcinogenicity presents another kind of problem. It is not only expensive but also time consuming to screen a single chemical. It requires, on an average three years, some 500 animals and more than half a million dollars in the USA. Besides, only a fraction of the available chemicals can be tested even in the technologically most advanced countries as the USA. A promising solution to the problem can be found in the use of cell culture systems from the experimental animals. Following exposure to a chemical, morphological changes indicative of carcinogenicity begin to appear in the cultured cells after about two to three weeks, and confirmation that altered cells can cause tumours in appropriate animals may require another four to six months. Cell culture systems from hamster and mouse have been effectively utilized for chemical tests, and other cell culture systems are also being developed. Exploitation of cell culture systems sharply reduces the time and the expense involved in screening, and offers opportunities of screening a large number of chemicals before marketing. Although these chemical carcinogen tests are generally applicable to humans, they may not always be perfect. Therefore, the ultimate test would be to screen chemicals for carcinogenicity using cell cultures derived from normal human cells. In this context, a great deal of effort has been made to refine the human cell culture system.

Short-term Prescreen of Chemicals

There are a number of short-term assays which are being currently utilized for screening the carcinogenicity of chemicals. These short-term procedures, which are mutagenicity assays, are based on the interaction of certain chemicals with DNA. Mutagen assays are being increasingly utilized as inexpensive prescreens of chemicals prior to testing in animal bioassays. There is a need to predict the carcinogenicity of chemicals before exposure to humans leads to cancer. One of the simplest methods for the prescreen of chemicals employs a mutant strain of the bacterium *Salmonella* that requires the amino acid histidine for its growth (the Ames test). This simply means that histidine-requiring *Salmonella* will only grow on a nutritional medium which contains histidine; the strain does not grow on a medium lacking histidine. The test consists of culturing the histidine-requiring bacterium on an agar plate containing: (a) a nutritional medium that fulfils every growth requirement except for histidine; (b) an extract from rat liver containing microsomal oxygenases for conversion of the suspected carcinogen to its active form; and (c) various quantities of the suspected chemical carcinogen. If the chemical under test can be converted into an active carcinogen (generally mutagen), then the mutagen so formed may cause backward mutation, that is, reversion to histidine-independent growth, and some of the bacteria will grow and form visible colonies on the agar plate. A positive correlation of 70 to 90 per cent has been found between mutagenicity in the short-term test and the carcinogenicity results of animal bioassays.

CHEMICAL CARCINOGENESIS: INITIATION AND PROMOTION

Most known chemical carcinogens can both promote and initiate neoplasms. These are known as complete carcinogens. A few chemicals can only initiate carcinogenesis in normal cells, but require another chemical for promotion leading to tumour formation. On the other hand, certain chemical agents can only promote cells, but cannot initiate the transformation process.

An important feature of most forms of carcinogenesis is the long latent period that elapses between the initial application of a carcinogen and the time of the first appearance of cancer. Another aspect of carcinogenesis is that the organism must be repeatedly exposed to the carcinogen for a sufficiently long time before the latter shows its effect. For example, a single application of coal tar does not lead to skin cancer in mouse; it is necessary to apply coal tar repeatedly to mouse skin for several months before any tumours become detectable. Cigarette smoke-associated lung cancer in humans may take some 10 to 15 years to develop. These and related observations on carcinogenesis have led to the generalization that relative to the life-span of an organism, whether mouse or human, the time course of carcinogenesis is invariably extraordinarily long.

Following the discovery that skin cancer could be produced by coal tar in various test animals, attempts were made to isolate and purify the active ingredients and to test them for carcinogenic potency. It was found that some of the constituents of tar were more carcinogenic, while others were more irritant. Although it is often possible to produce cancer in an animal by repeated application of a single chemical carcinogen, in certain situations, a sequential application of two substances is required for the production of tumours, suggesting that carcinogenesis may be separated into two distinct steps. These two major steps have been designated *initiation* and *promotion*. In one experiment, tumours were produced in mice by feeding them with a single dose of dimethybenzanthracene, DMBA (one of the active ingredients of coal tar), followed by a prolonged application to the skin of an irritant, croton oil. Tumours appeared on those regions of the skin where croton oil was repeatedly painted, but tumours failed to appear if the mice were not first fed with DMBA, or if the mice were first painted with croton oil and later fed with DMBA. This experiment shows that both ingredients are necessary for tumour production and they must be given in the following sequence: DMBA (initiator) and then croton oil (promoter). It would appear that the initiator produces a permanent, irreversible change in the mouse cells, and, subsequently, the promoter somehow provokes the tumour expression of initiated cells.

MECHANISMS OF CHEMICAL CARCINOGENESIS

Current cancer research has been directed towards elucidating the mechanisms involved in the transformation of a normal cell into a cancer cell. Chemical carcinogens may cause cancer in at least three ways. First, they may cause cancer by the direct modification of the genetic material, or by epigenetic changes involving alterations in the expression of the genetic material, but without accompanying alterations in its structure. Secondly, these chemicals may cause cancer by the activation of cancer-causing viruses. Thirdly, chemical carcinogens may initiate cancer through mutations (heritable changes) in the genetic material (DNA) of a cell. These mutations probably occur in the regulatory genes (suppressor genes), which, in some way, are essential for the orderly control of cell reproduction and cell differentiation. Or perhaps the mutations may occur in those suppressor genes which control the expression of cancer-inducing genes (proto-oncogenes) present in the genomes of multicellular organisms, including humans.

10

Environmental Factors and Cancer (IV)

RADIATION

Homo sapiens (human beings) have evolved, over millions of years, in spite of the exposure to cosmic and terrestrial radiation. And they will continue to live in this environment as long as the amounts of radiation do not exceed certain limits and become deadly. What amounts of radiation are safe for human existence? It has been estimated by the United Nations Scientific Committee on the Effects of Atomic Radiation that in the industrial countries the annual dose is about 240 mrem or 2.4 rad, and about 82 per cent of such radiation is from natural sources, including cosmic rays, terrestrial gamma-rays, radionuclides, and radon. The last source, radon, accounts for about 40 per cent of the total annual dose from homes and buildings built on radon-rich ground. Diagnostic and medical procedures account for about 17 per cent of the annual dose received by humans; however, the individual doses received may vary considerably, ranging from 1 to 3 rad annually.

There is considerable evidence to support the notion that both ionizing radiation (X-rays, gamma-rays) and non-ionizing radiation (ultraviolet rays) can cause cancer. In general, the physicians exposed to radiation, especially radiologists, are at a relatively higher risk of developing leukaemia compared to other physicians. However, the relative risk factor depends upon the dosage received by the radiologists during their professional career. Data on early radiologists, who started their profession in the 1920s, indicate that they faced a 10 times higher risk of dying from leukaemia than other physicians. This is because the early radiologists, not being aware of the radiation risk, inadvertently received large dosages of radiation (X-rays) themselves since they did not use adequate safety precautions to shield their bodies while X-raying their patients. On the other hand, radiologists who exercised greater precautions, showed only a small increase in the incidence of leukaemia as compared to other physicians. Nevertheless, chronic, repeated exposure to relatively small dosages of radiation of the order of 0.4 to 2 rad per week can increase the risk of leukaemia severalfold.

ATOMIC BOMBS AND CANCER

The tragic experiences of the Japanese atomic bomb survivors have provided us with the most convincing data that radiation causes cancer. In order to end the Second World War quickly, American planes dropped atomic bombs in August 1945 on two Japanese cities, Hiroshima and Nagasaki. The immediate effect of this atomic holocaust was tremendous human suffering. Those who were not incinerated in the terrible inferno of the blast fell victims to severe burns, destruction of bone marrow, diarrhoea, and hair loss. Persons who were not killed by the trauma of the blast showed 7 to 10 times higher incidence of leukaemia, and significantly increased rates of cancers of the breast, brain, bowel, and thyroid, as compared to the unexposed general population. Approximately 240,000 Japanese survivors had received radiation doses of 10 rad or more at a given time, a fact that enabled the determination of the latent periods and the onset of cancer and death. The populations of Hiroshima and Nagasaki who were exposed to the atomic explosion chiefly received gamma-rays, X-rays, and neutron type of radiation.

Among the various cancers, leukaemia was first detected in 1948 in the Japanese survivors who had received high doses of radiation, indicating that this cancer developed after a relatively short period of 2 to 3 years. The incidence of leukaemia reached a peak after 6 to 7 years (1951-52), and subsequently it declined slowly. The leukaemia death rate was significantly high among those survivors who had received radiation doses of 100 rad or more, even after 25 to 27 years (1970-72).

In the beginning of 1960, about 15 years after the bombing, it was observed that the mortality rate from cancers other than leukaemia increased considerably among the Japanese atomic bomb survivors who had received doses in excess of 100 rad. Different types of cancers developed among exposed children and adults. Cancers of the thyroid, brain, salivary gland, and the gastrointestinal system occurred more frequently among exposed children. On the other hand, cancers of the lung, breast, and the gastrointestinal system (but excluding stomach cancer) accounted for excess mortality among exposed adults. In general, individuals who were under 20 years of age at the time of the bombing seemed to have been particularly affected. Even almost half a century after the atomic blast, the Japanese are still dying of radiation-induced cancers.

NUCLEAR ACCIDENTS AND CANCER

An estimated 375 nuclear power plants are currently operational in the world. Another 150 are on order, and may become functional by the year 2000! This would mean that, by the turn of the century, an estimated 525 or more nuclear power plants, not to mention the nuclear-processing and research laboratories, may become operational worldwide. The nuclear power plants generate electricity based on a simple principle of nuclear fission. The fission of uranium 235 in the nuclear core produces a large amount of heat. This heat is transferred to the water surrounding the core and is utilized for producing enormous quantities of steam under pressure that drive the turbines for generating electricity.

Ever since these nuclear power plants went into operation in the 1950's, there has been fear of accidents, due to either human error or equipment malfunction. It is difficult to accurately catalogue all the nuclear power plant mishaps in the world with any precision, because many of these accidents have not been brought to the public notice. However, a number of nuclear power plant mishaps have been reported during the last several decades. Of these, two major nuclear power plant accidents have attracted global attention. The long-range effects of the fallout have been, and will continue to be, debated for a long time. The first occurred in 1979 at the Three-Mile Island, near Harrisburg, Pennsylvania, USA, and the second occurred at Chernobyl, near Kiev, in the former USSR in 1986. While there was a partial meltdown of the uranium fuel in the Three-Mile Island power plant, there was almost complete meltdown of the uranium fuel at the Chernobyl plant, spewing deadly radioactivity into the atmosphere.

Radioactive fallout from the Chernobyl disaster was detected in the European countries, in Japan, and in the USA. There were various types of radioactive particles in the fallout. Some of them decay very slowly (for example, strontium 90 and caesium 137), while others (for example, iodine 131) decay relatively quickly. The half-life of strontium 90 and caesium 137 is about 28 to 30 years (that is, every 28-30 years the radioactivity diminishes by half), while the half-life of iodine 131 is about 14 days. These long-lived and short-lived radioactive elements enter the food chain and pose health hazards for humans and animals. One of the long-range effects of radioactivity is the possibility of increasing the risk of cancer. In particular, foetuses and small children are highly vulnerable to the effects of radioactivity.

ULTRAVIOLET RADIATION AND RADIOACTIVE SUBSTANCES

Other forms of radiation, such as ultraviolet rays and radiation solutions (containing radium or thorium), are also known to be carcinogenic. Ultraviolet rays present in sunlight, which constitute non-ionizing radiation, have a low penetrating ability and have been causally related to the occurrence of skin cancer. Skin cancer occurs more frequently among sailors and farmers who spend long hours in bright sunlight. In those individuals constantly exposed to sunlight, skin cancer almost invariably occurs only in those body areas that are exposed to sunlight; skin cancer rarely occurs on body parts constantly covered by clothes.

The occupational tragedy involving the radium dial (in watches) painters is a grim reminder that exposure to any form of radioactivity can cause human cancer. The risk of bone cancer is greatly increased in persons who have ingested radium-containing solutions either occupationally or as medical therapy. Thorotrast, a radioactive substance (thorium oxide) used around the world between 1930 and 1950 as a contrast medium for diagnostic purposes, led to liver cancer and leukaemia in a significant number of patients who received it.

MAMMOGRAPHY

In the 1960s mammography was introduced as an aid for the early detection of breast cancer. The mammogram is a special X-ray of the soft tissue that uses lower energy radiation than for X-ray images of internal organs. When it was first introduced, it generated a great deal of enthusiasm that breast cancer deaths could be reduced substantially through early detection. However, recently some questions have been raised regarding mammography, especially whether the screening procedure is relatively safe for detection, or is it capable of inducing the breast cancer which it is supposed to detect. Over the past many years it has become clear that no level of radiation is absolutely safe, no matter how small the radiation dose may be. Therefore, every exposure to radiation entails a certain risk. But, sometimes, the circumstances justify the risk of exposure to radiation: for example, X-rays of a fractured bone, or chest X-rays of a person suspected to be suffering from tuberculosis. Likewise, mammography may be considered for screening women (between ages 35 and 50) who are at a higher risk of developing breast cancer because of the presence of lumps, thickening, chronic cystic mastitis, or a family history of breast cancer.

MICROWAVE RADIATION

Microwave radiation is given out by radar equipment and microwave ovens. Microwaves constitute non-ionizing radiation. They transmit their energy to biological systems, as heat produced, by causing the rapid oscillation of water and protein molecules in the cells. Although microwave radiation may cause some deleterious effects in the mammalian system, there is insufficient data on long-range effects and induction of cancer by microwaves.

THE EFFECT OF RADIATION ON CELLS

The effects of radiation on cells have been extensively investigated. The cells may be damaged by radiation in the following ways: (a) the damage may be in the form of cell killing; (b) chromosomal aberrations; or (c) gene mutations. The main target of radiation-induced damage, however, seems to be the genetic material – DNA. Normal cells have the ability to repair the damage inflicted by radiation, but when the damage is beyond the cell's ability to repair, it results in cell death.

Radiation may cause cancer by (a) inducing mutations (chromosomal aberrations or gene mutations) which may impair the suppressor genes that control the expression of cellular oncogenes, or activate the oncogenes themselves, and (b) inducing developmental changes.

Mutation and Cancer

A very frequent effect of radiation on cells is seen in the form of chromosome aberrations. These aberrations may involve chromosomal breaks, loss, addition, transfer of part of one chromosome to another (translocation), and inversion of segments within individual chromosomes. Some of these chromosome aberrations are not easily tolerated and may result in cell death because of loss of vital genetic information essential for cell survival. On the other hand, some of these chromosomal aberrations may be transmitted to the descendants of a progenitor cell in which such chromosome aberration(s) first arose without causing any loss of viability and the ability for normal cell reproduction, even though the genetic constitution of these cells has changed. Sometimes, some such cells may become cancerous because of loss over the control of cell reproduction and cell differentiation caused by chromosome loss, addition and/or rearrangement of specific genetic information in their cell genomes.

Radiation may also cause cancer by inducing gene mutations, not necessarily involving gross chromosomal abnormalities. Both ionizing radiation (X-rays, gamma-rays, neutrons) and non-ionizing radiation (ultraviolet rays) can cause gene mutations, even though the manner in which they cause a genetic change may differ. The main effect of the ultraviolet radiation is to produce 'dimers', that is, bonds between the adjacent bases in the DNA chain. If the dimers are correctly repaired, the cell behaves normally as though nothing ever happened. On the other hand, if a dimer is not properly repaired, it would invariably lead to mutation. Based on the fact that dimers being incorrectly repaired have a constant value in a cell, the mutation rate would be directly proportional to the dose of ultraviolet radiation.

The ionizing radiation (X-rays, neutrons) does not produce new bonds, but rather causes breaks in the DNA chain. X-rays produce single-chain breaks, and under normal circumstances, these breaks can be repaired by cellular enzymes. At least two independent hits, causing breaks in the opposite DNA chains, are necessary for a mutation to occur. Therefore, the mutation rate caused by X-rays increases as a square of the radiation dose. On the other hand, more energetic forms of radiation, for example, neutrons, commonly break both chains; that is, a single neutron hit can cause a mutation, and, therefore, the mutation rate increases proportionally to the dose. The data obtained on Japanese atomic bomb survivors substantiates this contention. The bomb dropped over Nagasaki produced mostly X-rays and the subsequent incidence of leukaemia in that city seems to be proportional to the square of the dose. On the other hand, the bomb over Hiroshima produced a great flux of neutrons, and the incidence of leukaemia in survivors in that city was directly proportional to the dose.

FORMS OF RADIATION AND CANCER

Certain forms of radiation produce tumours at specific sites, whereas others are capable of inducing a variety of different cancers. However, the response depends upon the form of radiation and the cell type of the host. For example, radium and radioactive strontium are generally deposited in the bone, and tend to produce bone cancer by irradiating bone cells. Similarly, radioactive iodine tends to produce thyroid cancer simply because iodine is deposited in the thyroid gland. Although ultraviolet radiation can cause damage to DNA of any cell type that is exposed to it, under normal circumstances, it is the skin cells that are directly exposed to ultraviolet rays in sunlight. Ultraviolet radiation, because of its low penetrating power, is only absorbed by the genetic material of the epidermal layers of the skin, and this radiation seems to be causally related to skin cancer by inducing damage (dimers) to DNA in skin cells.

The response to X-rays, on the other hand, is variable from one individual to another, or more precisely, from one tissue to another. On the whole, exposure to X-rays increases the risk of myeloid leukaemia and cancers of other organs; for example, breast, skin, and thyroid, suggesting that radiation carcinogenesis is a general biological phenomenon in all tissues. We are left with the puzzling situation that some tissues become cancerous, while others do not, following exposure to X-irradiation, even though radiation must be producing some kind of damage to cells in different tissues lying in its path. Since X-rays hit randomly at the genetic material, they may cause chromosome aberrations or gene mutations in cells of different tissues. As pointed out earlier, all sorts of genetic damage, however, do not lead to cancerous cells, but only some of the genetic lesions seem to have relevance to the origin of cancer. Consequently, the proneness of a cell type to cancer would ostensibly depend on its genetic constitution. This would suggest that different tissues may differ from each other with respect to certain genetic components. Such components may be the regulatory or suppressor genes that protect cells against cancer. Suppressor genes are tissue-specific and their state and number may differ in different tissues. By and large, the regulatory genes are diploid, that is, present as two normal copies in a tissue. However, variation from this diploid nature may occur due to impairment or loss of one copy of the regulatory gene, so that only one active copy of the gene is present (heterozygosity), or by doubling of the two active genes (duplication), or when multiple forms (redundancy), of the regulatory genes are present in different tissues. Whether a tissue would become cancerous or not following irradiation would depend on the active state of the tissue-specific suppressor genes: the lower the active number of suppressor genes' in a tissue, the greater the probability of its becoming cancerous. Loss or impairment of the suppressor genes' function in a specific tissue would invariably lead to activation of tissue-specific cellular oncogenes and to the origin of cancer in that tissue.

11

Viruses, Oncogenes, and Cancer

ONCOGENIC AND NON-ONCOGENIC VIRUSES

There are two types of viruses that cause diseases: the *oncogenic* viruses that are linked with cancer and *non-oncogenic* viruses which cause a wide variety of other diseases, such as small-pox, measles, mumps, polio, rabies and common colds. There are more than 100 different oncogenic viruses which have been shown to induce cancer in animals and plants. However, definitive proof that viruses cause cancer in humans is still lacking. That is not to say that viruses are not at all involved in the aetiology of human cancer, but rather that the kind of experimental approaches which have led to the evidence that viruses cause cancer in animals cannot be applied to humans for the simple reason that experimentally induced cancers are usually fatal to the test organism. Nevertheless, one of the most actively investigated areas of cancer research is the role of viruses and their oncogenes in the aetiology of human cancer. If a cause-and-effect relationship can be established between viruses and specific cancers, then it would offer an approach towards prevention and control of cancer through an immunization programme as practised for the other virally caused diseases, such as polio, small-pox, and measles.

The non-oncogenic viruses cause the disease by attacking/killing the cells of the tissue or organ they attack. However, they need not necessarily kill the organism as the body's immune systems are rapidly mobilized to fight the invading virus. The cells lost due to infection are rapidly replaced by cell reproduction. By contrast, oncogenic viruses do not generally kill the cells they infect, but somehow rather accelerate their cell reproduction. This leads to overcrowding of cells, failure of cells to mature, and loss of normal functioning of resulting cancer cells. Subsequently, the cancer cells may migrate to other parts of the body and may eventually cause the death of an organism. Human cancers strongly suspected of viral involvement include Burkitt's lymphoma, cervical cancer, liver cancer, and certain leukaemias. The oncogenic viruses are a heterogeneous group of unrelated viruses which have nothing in common in their structure and form. What is common to all oncogenic viruses is their inherent genetic capacity to induce cancer in a living cell, a genetic potential lacking in non-oncogenic viruses.

STRUCTURE AND REPRODUCTION OF VIRUSES

Viruses are extremely small entities, range from 20 to 250 mu, and their structure cannot be resolved by the light microscope but only by an electron microscope. Compared to a living cell, the viruses have a rather simple organization. The viruses contain a small chromosome that is made up of either DNA or RNA. The viral chromosome is tightly packed inside a protein coat which provides protection when the virus particle is outside a living cell. The viruses lead a dual existence: they are active and alive when they are within a living cell; they are inert when they are outside a living cell. The viruses can stay in the inert form in the air, water or soil for a long time. Viruses reproduce their progeny only when they are in a living cell. Once inside a living cell, the viral coat protein is stripped off and the viral chromosome uses the cell's machinery and material to make copies of its chromosome and many protein molecules for the viral coat. In nearly an hour after invading a living cell, a single virus particle produces hundreds of perfect copies of the original virus. Many viruses, particularly the non-oncogenic ones, rupture and kill the cells to release their progeny, which, in turn, invade new cells and start the viral reproduction cycle again, and in this way spread the infection in an organism. On the other hand, some viruses do not rupture the host cell to release the virus progeny. The newly formed virus particles pass through the cell membrane to the outside without apparently damaging the cell. These types of viruses generally do not kill the host cell, but instead use the cell as a long-term factory for the production of virus progeny.

How a normal cell gets converted into a cancer cell has not yet been clearly understood, but there is one aspect of the oncogenic viruses that distinguishes them from the physical and the chemical carcinogenic agents. The oncogenic viruses, in addition to initiating carcinogenesis, generally persist in the cancer cells and in their progeny (either as a free virus or in a 'hidden form') without necessarily killing the cells, and apparently contribute to the neoplastic expression of the cancerous growth. In contrast to this situation, the physical or chemical agents cause only the induction or promotion of cancer and play no further role thereafter. In other words, the continued presence of the carcinogen is not required for neoplastic development. Nevertheless, in both viral and physical or chemical carcinogenesis, the eventual emergence of cancer usually takes years or even decades, implying that additional changes are required for neoplastic development.

THE HOST RANGE OF VIRUSES

Following the discovery by Peyton Rous (in 1911) that viruses cause certain types of cancer in chicken, more than 100 different viruses have been found to be oncogenic in a variety of animals, including mice, rats, rabbits, hamsters, dogs, and monkeys. With the exception of a few viruses, most others produce cancer only in particular types of animals. For example, viruses that cause cancer in mice may not be able to do so when injected in chicken, or those which cause cancer in rats may not produce tumours in monkeys. It seems that most oncogenic viruses tend to restrict their oncogenic activity to a particular animal host. So far none of the viruses that cause cancer in animals has been found to be oncogenic in humans.

A number of viruses have been studied using animal systems for an understanding of how a virus transforms a normal cell into a cancer cell. Although we still do not precisely know how a virus works towards converting a normal cell, detailed investigations of specific oncogenic viruses in experimental animals have provided several useful leads. All the major types of cancer that occur in humans can be produced in the test animals by some 100 oncogenic viruses. Although most carcinogenic viruses operate in a restricted host range and usually cause cancer in a single organ in a particular animal, at least a few of these viruses are capable of producing more than one kind of cancer in several different animals. The polyoma virus (DNA virus), first discovered as a causal agent for the cancer of salivary gland in mouse, is one such multipotential virus. Subsequently, polyoma virus was found not only to cause tumours in many different tissues of mouse, but also to induce tumours in several different animals, including rats, hamsters and guinea pigs. However, the polyoma virus does not appear to cause cancer in humans.

DNA TUMOUR VIRUSES

A few DNA viruses have been linked to some human cancers. These include the Epstein-Barr virus associated with lymphomas and nasopharyngeal cancer, hepatitis B virus with liver cancer, and human papilloma virus with cervical and other genital cancers in women.

The Epstein-Barr Virus

In 1958 Burkitt reported the discovery of a strange new disease among children in Uganda, East Africa, which caused the swelling of the jaws and the lymphoid tissue. This disease was later identified as malignant lymphoma, composed of undifferentiated lymphoblasts, and was named after the discoverer, Burkitt. Although the incidence of Burkitt's lymphoma is the highest in tropical Africa and Papua New Guinea, sporadic cases of this disease have been reported from different countries throughout the world. Burkitt's lymphoma occurs predominantly in children between the ages of two and 14, with a peak incidence at seven years. A member of the herpesvirus group called the Epstein-Barr virus (EBV) (Fig. 11.1) has been found to be associated with Burkitt's lymphoma, and is suspected to be causal in this disease. A specific chromosome aberration involving a translocation of a specific region of chromosome 8 (carrying a cellular oncogene, *c-myc*) to chromosome 14 has been observed in a majority of Burkitt's lymphoma patients. Whether or not the Epstein-Barr virus causes a specific mutation involving a translocation of the cellular oncogene *c-myc* to new location, thereby causing position effect leading to the onset of lymphoma, remains an intriguing possibility. However, it seems that some additional genetic/developmental changes may be necessary for the malignant transformation in Burkitt's lymphoma.

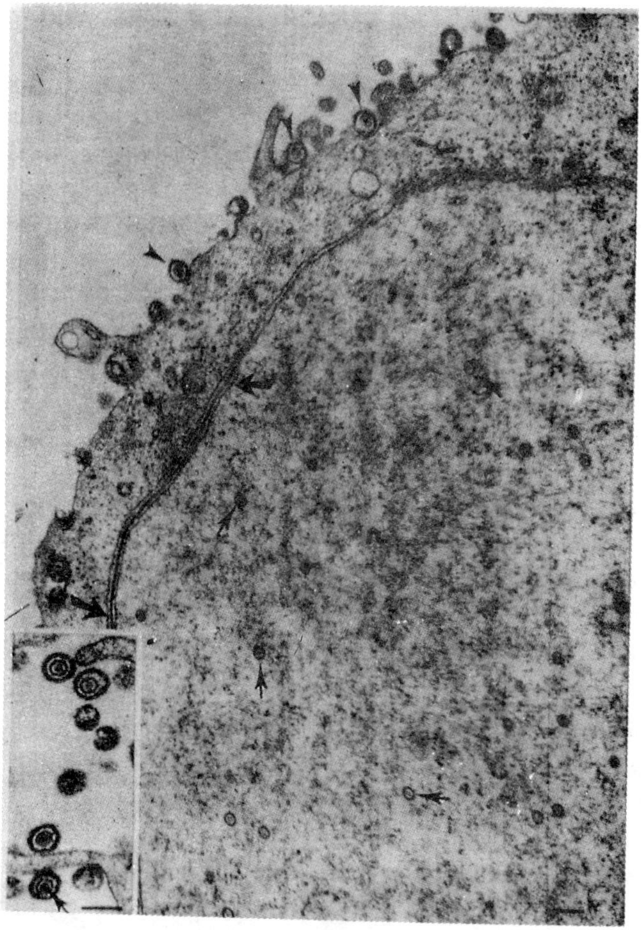

Fig. 11.1 This section of a cell is from a Burkitt's lymphoma cell line producing the Epstein-Barr virus (EBV) Nuleocapsids (thin arrows) with cores of low density are present in the nucleus (n); reduplication of the nuclear membrane (thick arrows) and extracellular virus particles (arrowheads). *Inset*: extracellular virus particles consisting of a nucleocapsid surrounded by an envelope, one of them (arrow) shows a nucleocapsid with a dense core. Bar represents 200 nm. (*Courtesy*: Dr. Jero Calafat, The Netherlands Cancer Institute, Amsterdam.)

The Hepatitis B Virus

Epidemiological studies have shown that the hepatitis B virus has become widespread in South-east Asia and, especially, in southern China. In these regions more than 300 million people have become long-term carriers of the hepatitis B virus. It has been observed that the carriers of this virus run a risk of developing liver cancer *at least* 100 times greater than the non-carriers. The hepatitis B virus can be transmitted horizontally as well as vertically. Insufficient hygiene and intimate contacts with carriers of hepatitis B virus lead to horizontal spread of the virus in the population. The vertical route (non-hereditary) of viral transmission takes place from the carrier mother to her offspring at birth. Effective control against hepatitis B infection includes immunization by vaccines that have been developed since 1980.

The Human Papilloma Virus

Certain strains of the human papilloma virus have been linked to cancers of the cervix and genitalia in women. However, only a small proportion of women infected with the human papilloma virus develop cervical cancer. It appears that the infection of women with this virus may also be insufficient to cause cancer. However, some other factors may also be involved. The human papilloma virus in appropriate genotypes may activate cellular oncogene(s) to initiate carcinogenesis, and that additional changes would be necessary for the development of cervical cancer. On the other hand, in a great majority of women infected with the human papilloma virus, certain cellular interfering factors may inhibit the expression of transforming genes, or immune surveillance mechanisms involving natural killer cells may act as the mediators in developing cellular immunity against human papilloma virus-related cancers.

RNA TUMOUR VIRUSES

There are several other cancer-inducing viruses which contain RNA instead of DNA as their genetic material. A number of RNA viruses, called retroviruses, have been shown to induce cancer in a variety of animals such as mouse, rat, cat, chicken, turkey, hamster, guinea pig, rabbit, dog and cow, and also in subhuman primates. Certain retroviruses have been implicated in the aetiology of some human cancers.

Retroviruses and Oncogenes

Retroviruses are a group of RNA viruses that are unique in their mode of replication and transmission of genetic material. Some of the retroviruses are highly oncogenic. These viruses are capable of transforming cells *in vitro* and induce tumours in animals. The retroviruses replicate by reverse 'transcription' (flow of genetic information from RNA to DNA) via a DNA provirus that can integrate into cellular DNA. The acute transforming retroviruses seem to have acquired their oncogenes from the cellular proto-oncogenes of animals, including humans, by a process called transduction (acquisition). The cellular proto-oncogenes, also called cellular oncogenes (c-*onc*), are normal cellular genes, and have been so termed because, by transduction into retroviruses, they have been shown to be oncogenic in animals. It seems that oncogenes were not present in the ancestral retroviruses, but these genes were picked up by the viruses during their transition from the non-transforming form to the oncogenic virus. Each retrovirus strain carries a single oncogene, gained from animal or human cellular genes. It seems highly likely that during transduction the cellular proto-oncogene captured by the retrovirus is subsequently modified by a genetic change or changes (mutation or mutations) to create a viral oncogene. Approximately 100 cellular oncogenes have been characterized; of these only 20 identified by their presence in the retroviruses are presented in Table 11.1.

Table 11.1 Transforming genes of oncogenic retroviruses and their location on human chromosomes. (*Source*: M. Park and G.F. Vande Woude, in: *Cancer -- Principles and Practices of Oncology*, edited by V.T. De Vita *et al.*, third edition, 1989; modified.)

Retrovirus	*Species of origin*	*Oncogene*	*Location on human chromosome*
Rous' sarcoma	Chicken	*src*	20
Avian myeloblastosis	Chicken	*myb*	6q22-24
Avian myelocytomatosis	Chicken	*myc*	8q24
Avian erythroblastosis	Chicken	*erb* A	17p11-q21
Avian erythroblastosis	Chicken	*erb* B	7
Avian SK770	Chicken	*ski*	1
Abelson leukaemia	Mouse	*abl*	9q34
FBJ osteosarcoma	Mouse	*fos*	2
Murine sarcoma	Mouse	*raf* 1	3p25
Murine sarcoma	Mouse	*raf* 2	4
Moloney murine sarcoma	Mouse	*mos*	8q22
Harvey murine sarcoma	Rat	H-*ras* 1	11p14
Harrvey murine sarcoma	Rat	H-*ras* 2	X
Kirsten murine sarcoma	Rat	K-*ras* 1	6
Kirsten murine sarcoma	Rat	K-*ras* 2	12
Feline sarcoma	Cat	*fms*	5q34
Reticuloendotheliosis	Turkey	*rel*	2p11
Simian sarcoma	Woolly monkey	*sis*	22
None	Human	N-*ras*	1p32
None	Human	N-*myc*	2

Replication and Oncogenic Transformation

The RNA genome of the retroviruses is wrapped in a core of viral protein. The core, in turn, is surrounded by an envelope covered with viral glycoproteins derived from the membrane of the previous host cell. Retroviruses get attached to cells with the help of normal cell surface proteins which are specifically recognized by viral envelope proteins and enter the cell by an invagination mechanism called 'endocytosis'. The cells have evolved the same mechanism for ingestion of beneficial extracellular substances such as growth factors. Following entry into the cell, an enzymatically active nucleoprotein complex, derived from the envelope, initiates reverse transcription of RNA into DNA and integration of the provirus into the host genome. Once the retroviral genome becomes part of the host genome, the provirus becomes dependent on its host for replication of new retroviral particles, although several cellular functions are regulated by viral signals.

The retrovirus RNA encodes for three genes, referred to as *gag*, *pol*, and *env*. The *gag* and *env* genes encode for structural proteins necessary for a virion frame, while the *pol* gene seems to provide enzymes for reverse transcriptase and integration of the proviral DNA sequences in the host genome.

Oncogenic retroviruses isolated from vertebrates such as fish, chickens, rodents, cats, subhuman primates and humans, generally induce sarcomas (tumours of mesenchymal origin, i.e., mesodermal embryonal tissue), various kinds of leukaemias, but less frequently epithelial malignancies (the most common human cancers), including carcinomas of the breast, kidney and liver.

The oncogenic retroviruses seem to fall into two broad groups. One typified by the Rous sarcoma virus (RSV) and referred to as acute transforming retroviruses, which carry oncogenes, can produce tumours in newborn animals in less than two weeks. The second group, typified by leukaemia and leukosis retroviruses, lack the oncogenes, and do not transform cells in culture, but produce tumours in animals after a relatively long latent period (more than three months), most probably by allowing the frequency integration of the retrovirus adjacent to cellular oncogenes.

The retroviruses can integrate at many sites in the host chromosomes. Such proviral integration may interfere with various cellular functions. The insertion of provirus sequences next to regulatory genes may impair regulatory gene function by mutation or position effect, which, in turn, could lead to abnormal activity of the structural genes, including cellular oncogenes. The retroviruses that cause leukaemia in animals have been isolated from humans, and these are known as human T-cell leukaemia viruses (HTLV). At least one of the T-cell leukaemias in humans may be linked to these types of retroviruses.

It has been shown that nearly all the known viral oncogenes (v-*onc*) have been derived from normal cellular genes, the so-called cellular oncogenes (c-*onc*), also known as proto-oncogenes. This implies that certain genetic changes are required in the control and/or expression of the cellular oncogenes to initiate carcinogenesis. The v-*onc* genes derived from vertebrate cells may not necessarily contain complete genetic information present in the c-*onc*. The genetic information unessential for neoplastic transformation may be deleted in the v-*onc* during transduction from the c-*onc*. Therefore, the v-*onc* of certain retroviruses, for example, v-*src* and v-*mos*, may differ from its progenitor c-*onc*, in terms of its genetic constitution, reflected by the composition of amino acids. These amino acids may or may not be essential for cellular transformation. However, most of the v-*onc* and c-*onc* genes have sufficient genetic homology to substantiate their origin. In contrast, certain retroviruses, including those involved in leukaemia and mammary tumour, apparently do not carry the vertebrate oncogenes but are capable of inducing neoplasms in test animals. One such retrovirus is the mouse mammary tumour virus (MMTV).

Mouse Mammary Tumour Virus

The mouse mammary tumour virus (MMTV), also known as the Bittner virus (named after its discoverer), has been shown to be involved in mammary gland cancer in mice. The virus is commonly transmitted to the offspring through mother's milk, and only infects the female mice. The development of mammary cancer is, however, dependent upon a complex interplay among the virus, the genetic constitution of the host and the hormonal factors. All these three factors determine whether or not mammary cancer will develop in a certain strain of mice. In one inbred strain (C3H) there are certain colonies of mice in which the incidence of mammary cancer is exceedingly high and may affect 95 to 100 per cent of the female animals. The females in such strains have a very large amount of infectious virus particles in their milk.

In contrast, there are 'low mammary cancer' strains of mice, in which only a small percentage of the females ever develop the disease. That the MMTV plays a very important role in the development of mammary cancer has been clearly demonstrated by allowing the newborn female mice from the 'low mammary cancer' strain to be foster-nursed by mothers from the 'high mammary cancer' strain. These foster-nursed female mice develop high incidences of mammary cancer when they reach adulthood. On the other hand, when newborn female mice from the 'high mammary cancer' strain are foster-nursed by mothers from a 'low mammary cancer' strain, the incidenc of mammary tumours are dramatically low or absent in these foster-nursed female mice. These experiments clearly demonstrate that mammary cancer in mice is a communicable disease and MMTV can be most effectively transmitted to the offspring through mother's milk.

In another strain of mouse (C3HfB), the mammary cancer virus called NIV (nodule-inducing virus) is transmitted through the males and females as a provirus via the germline, but this virus does not seem to be transmitted through the milk. There exists a third kind of model in mice (the GR strain) where the virus is readily transmitted through both males and females; it can also be communicated via the milk. To summarize, there are at least three models for the transmission of mammary cancer in mice: (1) the virus is primarily transmitted through the milk; (2) the virus is transmitted through male and female mice (through germline), but not through the milk; and (3) the virus is transmitted through male and females (through germline) and also through the milk.

Is a Virus Involved in the Aetiology of Human Breast Cancer?

The studies on mammary cancer in mice have raised certain important questions regarding breast cancer in human females. Is a virus involved in the complex aetiology of human breast cancer? If yes, how is it transmitted from mothers to daughters? Does the human milk contain any virus particles? If so, are such virus particles similar or dissimilar to those found in the mouse mammary cancer? Has breast feeding any effect on human breast cancer? Whether or not a specific retrovirus or oncogene plays an important role in the aetiology of human breast cancer is not clear at the present time.

It has been observed that breast cancer seems to run in certain families. There are some families with a high incidence of breast cancer, and there are others having a low or almost zero incidence of this disease. This implies that there is a tendency to inherit breast cancer in certain families, and this inherited susceptibility may in part determine whether a certain woman would develop breast cancer or not. In addition to the inherited susceptibility, it is possible that, as in the case of mice, additional information may be brought in by a certain virus, which may be required for the development of human breast cancer. In fact, virus-like particles have been discovered in the milk of certain women, particularly in the Parsi women of India and also in Western women with a high incidence of breast cancer. The presence of virus-like particles in the human breast milk is intriguing. This leads us to the next question. Does breast feeding have any effect on human breast cancer?

There are two ways of looking at this question. One is whether breast feeding a baby minimizes the risk of breast cancer in the mothers? The results of careful investigations have revealed that there is no direct relationship between breast feeding and the infliction of breast cancer. The second aspect which is more relevant to our present discussion is the fact that mothers with a history of breast cancer in their families may transmit the virus-like particles (if eventually proven to be the cause of breast cancer) to their female children by breast feeding them. Therefore, nursing in those cases may increase the risk of breast cancer in the female offspring. However, at the present time, it is not certain whether the virus-like particles in the milk are causally related to human breast cancer.

The Leukaemia Virus

Numerous viruses have been shown to induce different types of leukaemias in a variety of animals. Leukaemia viruses have been extensively investigated in mice. As in mammary cancer of mice, there are 'high leukaemic' and 'low leukaemic' strains of mice. In other words, only animals with a certain genetic constitution develop leukaemia. For a long time it was not known how the animals, particularly mice, become infected with leukaemia. In certain strains of mice leukaemia can be induced by certain leukaemic viruses, while, in other strains, leukaemia develops spontaneously, apparently without the introduction of the viruses by experimental means. In these later strains leukaemia viruses are generally present without necessarily causing leukaemia, and these viruses are transmitted from parents to offspring through the egg and sperm cells. Leukaemia develops in these strains when the leukaemic virus present in the dormant form in the mouse cells is apparently activated by certain agents, such as chemicals, radiation, or an environmental stress. The leukaemic viruses isolated from certain strains of mice can also induce leukaemia in other strains of mice or rats, when these viruses are injected into newborn or very young animals. The leukaemic viruses seem to be less effective in inducing leukaemia when they are injected into older animals. So here is an example of viruses that are not only leukaemic to the host of their origin, but also induce leukaemia when injected into related or even unrelated animals.

Types of Human Leukaemias

Different types of leukaemias have also been extensively investigated in human beings. Leukaemias are cancers of certain cell types, particularly the white blood cells (leucocytes and lymphocytes). The normal function of the white blood cells is to provide defence against bacterial and viral infections. In leukaemias, by contrast, the precursor cells of the white blood cells do not differentiate and mature, but instead proliferate into functionless, immature cells which interfere with the normal functioning of the blood. Leukaemias are named after the cell type of their origin: acute myeloblastic leukaemia, derived from the myeloblast cells of the bone marrow which do not differentiate and mature into leucocytes; acute lymphoblastic leukaemia, derived from the lymphoblast cells of the lymphoid tissue which do not mature into lymphocytes; and chronic myeloid or granulocytic leukaemia, derived from the bone marrow cells of the circulating blood. Leukaemias generally afflict young children, but may also develop in adults and are relatively less common in older individuals.

Viruses and Human Leukaemia

Several studies have suggested that certain leukaemia viruses (retroviruses) may be involved in the aetiology of human leukaemias. Subviral particles to complete viral particles have been detected in the blood samples from leukaemic patients. Suggestions have been made that leukaemia viruses may have been communicated to humans through contact with household pets, such as cats, which harbour a leukaemia virus, FeLV (feline leukaemia virus) that spreads as an infectious agent from one cat to another, or from the primates. And once this virus enters a human being, it could be transmitted with or without an intermediate virus in the human populations. Nevertheless, definitive proof concerning viral involvement in human leukaemia is still lacking.

AIDS

AIDS (acquired immunodeficiency syndrome) is a deadly disease that destroys the body's defence (immune) system. An intact immune system is necessary and essential for combating infections. There is substantial evidence to suggest that AIDS is caused by a retrovirus called HIV (human immunodeficiency virus). When the AIDS virus invades the immune system T cells (T for thymus, a class of lymphocytes known as helper cells), the viral RNA is transcribed 'backwards' into DNA by a viral enzyme called reverse transcriptase. The viral DNA is spliced into the DNA of the host cell. The integrated virus DNA then instructs the cell's reproductive machinery to replicate AIDS virus particles, which emerge from the host cell and infect new cells. In this way, the deadly virus destroys the T lymphocytes and also the body's defence against other infections. As the disease progresses, AIDS symptoms appear, including swollen lymphnodes, multiple bacterial and viral infections, dementia (brain cell damage), and secondary cancers, years after the first contact with the AIDS virus.

AIDS cases have been reported worldwide. According to a recent World Health Organization (WHO) report, more than 13 million people have become infected with the AIDS virus, and it has been estimated that by the year 2000 some 40 million inhabitants of Planet Earth may become victims of this pandemic. Nowhere is AIDS more widespread than in Africa. WHO estimates that more than 8 million persons are already infected with the AIDS virus in subSahara Africa. In the United States of America an estimated 1 million young people and adults are infected with HIV. AIDS was initially ascribed in the early 1980s to the 'gay' population of the USA, since most of the victims of the disease were homosexual men. For a while, it was thought that AIDS afflicts males more frequently than females, since in the USA. male victims outnumbered their female counterparts by a wide margin. But this turned out to be a wrong conclusion.

As more attention was paid to AIDS victims in Africa and Haiti (a possible route of the AIDS virus to the USA), it became clear that the disease strikes both males and females in approximately equal numbers. As it turns out, there is a large 'gay' population in the USA, and the homosexual male group was the first to be infected by the AIDS virus, and the 'gays' spread the disease among themselves. By contrast, homosexuality is rather uncommon in African countries, yet the AIDS virus is widespread in the population. Therefore, AIDS is not a homosexual disease. It strikes both sexes in all age groups and races, and has become widespread via heterosexual intercourse. In other words, the AIDS virus can be transmitted horizontally as likely from males to females, or vice versa.

The AIDS virus is transmitted by intimate sex, contaminated needles (used by drug addicts), blood transfusion (in case the blood is contaminated by HIV), and by infection at birth. The danger of horizontal transmission to healthy individuals is restricted, not only from the AIDS patients, but also from carriers of the AIDS virus, who apparently show no symptoms of the disease. Some persons in the population remain unaffected by the disease, even though they carry HIV. This might suggest a genetic susceptibility to AIDS.

The therapy against AIDS has posed a difficult problem. Several anti-viral drugs are being tested for treatment against AIDS. These include AZT (azidothymidine), ddI (Videx), and pyridinone. As yet there is no effective vaccine for curing or controlling AIDS, but several biotechnological and pharmaceutical companies are working on the development of one. Hopefully, there is only one major type of virus involved in AIDS and not different variants of HIV, or more than one retrovirus. The latter possibility might complicate therapeutic and control strategies directed towards AIDS.

TRANSFORMATION OF CELLS BY VIRUSES

Although viruses have been shown to induce cancer in animals and are actively pursued for their possible role in human cancer, it is far from clear how viruses transform normal cells into cancer cells. It has been shown that following infection by an oncogenic virus, the viral genetic material becomes attached at certain location(s) in the cellular DNA. Following integration of viral genetic information in the host genome, the viral gene or genes replicates or replicate along with cellular DNA, before the cell begins division, and is subsequently transmitted to the descendants of the original cell in which the viral gene was integrated. It appears that continuous retention of the viral genetic information is necessary for the maintenance of the cancerous state. Beyond the integration of viral genetic information in the DNA of a cell, it is not clear as to what is the precise mechanism of transformation of a normal cell into a cancer cell by virtue of this addition of the viral genetic information. There are at least three possible ways by which viruses might transform normal cells: (1) a certain segment of the viral chromosome containing the cancer information (oncogene) acts as a template for the production of new and specific substances required for the transformation of normal cells into cancer cells and for maintenance of the cancerous state; (2) the viral gene products do not act directly to transform cells, but do so indirectly by bringing about activation, on a continuous basis, of those cellular genes that are involved in cell division and growth; and (3) the viruses might act as carcinogens or cocarcinogens and cause defects in certain tissue-specific genes, particularly regulatory genes, that normally prevent the expression of cellular oncogenes.

Regardless of the mechanism(s) of transformation, one of the first cellular functions associated with viral infection is the activation of the biosynthetic machinery of the cell geared towards synthesis of chromosomal DNA, proteins and enzymes for cell reproduction, and this reproduction capacity of the cancer cells is maintained in a persistent momentum throughout the development of the cancerous state. The cells transformed by an oncogenic virus have a new protein, the so-called 'tumour antigen' or simply 'T antigen', on their surface. The presence of T antigen serves as an indicator of a specific viral involvement in a specific type of cancer. Current evidence suggests that T antigen seems to play an important role in the initiation and maintenance of the transformed state. Another indicator of the viral involvement in cancer is the presence of a specific enzyme called 'reverse transcriptase', which is an RNA-dependent DNA polymerase involved in the translation of viral RNA into DNA in the cells transformed by RNA tumour viruses. Although reverse transcriptase is commonly associated with RNA virus-transformed cells, it has been occasionally recovered from certain normal cells. Typically, reverse transcriptase is detectable in animal tumours induced by RNA tumour viruses. However, this enzyme has also been detected in human leukaemia and breast cancer. The reverse transcriptase from these human cancers shows relatedness to the reverse transcriptase isolated from certain RNA viruses associated with leukaemia in baboon (for human leukaemia), and mammary cancer in mouse and monkey (for human breast cancer). This may also possibly indicate the route of infection for leukaemia and mammary tumour viruses from these animals to humans, but may not be necessarily involved in the causation of leukaemia or breast cancer in humans.

12

Aging and Cancer

Although cancer can occur in individuals at any age, from childhood through adulthood, it is predominantly a disease of old age. The incidence of most cancers increases dramatically with age. For example, the cancer of the large intestine increases more than 100-fold between the ages of 30 and 80. The question then arises: is there any relationship between aging and cancer? Are older people particularly more vulnerable to cancer attack? Before we attempt to answer these questions, let us first examine what is meant by aging.

WHAT IS AGING?

Aging is a time-related process. It is a natural process that occurs in all living beings. Aging occurs at different rates in different species. For example, a mouse reaches old age at about 2 years, a dog at 12 years, a human at 60 years, and an elephant at 70 years, and a Galapagos tortoise at 150 years. These figures are approximations, and there is a fluctuation around these average values. This means that aging also progresses at different rates among individuals of a species. This, again, suggests that both aging rates and the aging process are, to a large extent, under genetic control. However, the aging rate may be subjected to change by the environmental factors, including diet, pollutants, and radiation. At the end of the aging process the individual dies. We do not know what really causes aging. But some insight into the aging process has been gained by cell culture studies.

By employing human fibroblast cells, L. Hayflick showed that they have a finite life span in culture. Fibroblast cultures derived from embryonic lung cells undergo about 50 divisions before they die. On the other hand, fibroblasts from adult lung cells reach senescence after about 20 divisions and then they die. Certain cell lines from the rat have been maintained in culture for over 100 doublings. It would appear that the life span may be dependent upon the cell type, the donor species, and the culture conditions. Numerous studies on cells/tissues taken from whole animals have shown that total activity of a number of enzymes changes with age. This might suggest that mutations might accumulate as tissues age. One theory has it that aging is an end result of cellular mutations that have occurred throughout the life of an organism, and that such mutations affect the normal functioning and viability of the cells as they age. Another model on aging proposed by L.E. Orgel called the 'error catastrophe' hypothesis assumes that as cells age they tend to be more error-prone in their protein synthesis and these errors accumulate in the tissues as they age. The frequency of errors of protein synthesis increases rapidly as cells age and then they finally die. According to another school of thought, aging is an end result of a predetermined developmental genetic programme in each species, which may not necessarily require the accumulation of mutations or errors of protein synthesis. This programme is subject to environmental influences, which may modify the rate of aging in an individual. Yet another postulate has it that aging is a byproduct of an evolutionary process, in which many genes with immediate survival value are selected by nature, but on a long-range basis, the same genes have deleterious consequences. In other words, action and expression of many genes are subject to change in space and time. Some of the free radicals/chemicals produced by the body may be useful against bacterial or viral functions, but the same chemicals may also contribute to DNA damage. Some of these chemicals, for example, oxidants, known as endogenous mutagens, that may cause a genetic change, will accumulate in the body and may contribute to aging and cancer. Whatever the nature of the aging process, definite changes occur in different tissues of the body. One of the easily recognized signs of old age in humans is the loss of elasticity of the skin. Along with external changes, a number of other changes also occur in all the cells of the body.

All the cells in the body have a definite life span. For example, the life span of a red blood cell is about 120 days, while that of the cells lining the intestine may be one or two days. Likewise, the tissues and organs in the body seem to have a limited life span. Although different organs in the body may attain senescence at different times, failure of any one of the vital organs during the senescence phase may result in the death of an individual. This does not mean that the failure of an organ does not occur before senescence; failure can occur at any time due to a number of causes that interfere with the normal functioning of an organ. The performance of most tissues and organs is far below optimal during senescence. The individual becomes more susceptible to the attack of infectious diseases due to poor functioning of the immune tissues. Since cancer is a disease of old age, it has been suggested that cancer is one facet of the overall aging programme. Sometimes, it is stated with fatalistic resignation that man is destined to die of diseases peculiar to old age, such as cancer or heart disease.

ASSOCIATION BETWEEN AGING AND CANCER

Although the process of aging and development of cancer seem to be related, it is possible that aging and cancer are associated processes running a parallel course. This would imply that different sets of genes may be involved in the two processes, that is, genes involved in the control of the aging process are quite different from those involved in the prevention of cancer development. Most cancer cells are clonal (single cell) in origin, and therefore might have arisen as a result of mutational events, following gene-environment interactions. On the other hand, aging, even though influenced by environmental factors, seems to be a more programmed and directed process. Since most cancers develop after a long latent period extending from 5 to 20 years, it would appear that the total cancer experience is a result of a series of steps that have been initiated long before the clinical symptoms of the disease are recognized, and in most common cancers that seems to happen when one has attained old age.

13

The Origin of Cancer

It is now recognized that both genetic and environmental factors play an important role in the aetiology of cancer. Epidemiological data suggest that a majority of human cancers are strongly influenced by environmental factors, such as chemical carcinogens, radiation, ultraviolet rays, asbestos, tobacco smoke, and diet. Viruses have also been implicated in the aetiology of some human cancers. In addition, inherited predisposition is known to exist for a number of human cancers. Obviously, there is a multiplicity of diverse factors that seem to be involved in the causation of cancer. For example: tobacco smoke seems to be causally related to lung cancer, nitrosoamines to stomach cancer and dietary animal fat to colonic cancer. This might suggest that there may be several different basic mechanisms that are triggered off by diverse environmental factors for the *origin* of different human cancers. Although there might be some variation in the way a normal cell initially interacts with a particular environmental factor before it is transformed into a cancer cell, there is lack of evidence to support the suggestion that there are several different basic mechanisms for the origin of cancer. Regardless of what causes cancer, it appears that the end result of the transformation is nearly the same, namely, unrestrained cell reproduction usually accompanied by aberrant cell differentiation. This would imply that transformation of a normal cell to a cancer cell presumably affects common cellular genetic mechanism(s) which seems to be critical for cell reproduction and differentiation. Since the daughter cells exhibit properties similar to the progenitor cancer cell, and since cell heredity is maintained through subsequent cell reproductions, cancer is generally believed to be a genetic disease involving defects at the biochemical and molecular levels. Although the precise nature of the mechanism(s) for transformation of normal cell to a cancer cell is not yet fully understood, it seems probable that diverse environmental factors, singly or in combination, may, in a great majority of cases, directly or indirectly affect the genetic components of the cell, particularly the regulatory genes or 'suppressor genes', by causing certain genetic changes (gene mutations or chromosome abnormalities) and/or inducing an epigenetic (developmental) change. Major concepts for the origin of cancer are presented as follows.

THE MUTATION CONCEPT

The mutation concept of cancer is indeed an old one and goes back to the beginning of the present century. In 1914 Theodore Boveri published a book entitled *Zur Frage der Entstehung maligner Tumoren* (*On the Origin of Malignant Tumours*). Boveri mentioned in the introduction of his book that he was writing on the tumour problem as a zoologist, and that he had not really worked on any special area of tumour research. Nevertheless, Boveri's keen observations, comments on cell biology, and hypothesis on the origin of tumours have had a profound influence on modernday cancer research. Boveri commented that: (a) tumour cells are derived from normal cells, and causes of abnormalities are inherent in the tumour cells; and (b) cells of malignant tumours have a cellular defect, having lost part of the normal cellular component(s). Boveri further postulated that the abnormal morphology of chromosomes (in particular the chromotin complex) frequently observed in tumour cells was central to the origin of tumours. Since that time, of course, it has been established that chromosomes are the carriers of genes made up of the hereditary substance DNA. Boveri's concept of the abnormal chromatin complex in tumour cells, which has come to be known as the *somatic mutation theory of cancer,* has been widely discussed in relation to physical and chemical carcinogenesis. However, the manner by which mutations produce malignancy is still conjectural. Carcinogens interact with, and cause damage to, DNA. If this damage is not repaired properly, it is fixed as a mutation in the replicating DNA molecule. Mutations affecting the genes involved in the regulation of cell reproduction and differentiation may lead to neoplastic development.

Recent genetic theories of carcinogenesis have invoked the concept that sites of mutation are the regulatory or suppressor genes that normally control the expression of genetic information, which when uncontrolled, leads to neoplastic development. Such genetic information may be encoded by multiple structural genes, the so-called transforming (*Tr*), or tumour (*Tu*) genes, or more recently cellular oncogenes (c-*onc*), and some of these genes may be tissue-specific. The precise function of these genes remains conjectural. However, it may be supposed that these potentially cancer-causing genes are transiently active during different stages of embryonic development. Those genes that accomplish the necessary regulation of this potentially tumour-inducing information are designated as 'regulatory genes' (*R*-genes) and their location as 'regulatory loci'. Regulatory loci are specific for a given tissue or cell type, and the number of such loci may differ for different tissues. Elimination of particular *R*-genes or impairment of the *R*-gene function by environmental factors, such as radiation or chemical carcinogens, release the *onc*-genes from their normal constraint and trigger off a chain of events which may lead to the development of tissue-specific neoplasms.

THE EPIGENETIC CONCEPT

The underlying implication of the epigenetic (or developmental) concept is that cancer need not be mutational in origin, but could be due to epigenetic changes. The prevalent thesis is that development and differentiation are the result of epigenetically controlled changes in the expression of various genes, and not the result of changes in the structure of the genes. Likewise, cancer, which is characterized by defects in differentiation, may be the result of epigenetic changes in the expression of genes and not due to a change (mutation) in the primary structure of the genetic material. According to this line of thinking, cancer would be potentially reversible. The differentiation hypothesis does not invoke the presence of specific cancer genes, but instead considers that certain genes normally involved in cell reproduction and tissue differentiation, when misprogrammed, may lead to neoplastic development.

THE VIRAL CONCEPT

Viruses have been shown to induce tumours in animals, and have been implicated in the aetiology of some human cancers. Some scientists have proposed that the cancer-causing genetic information, the viral oncogenes, may be present in the cells of higher organisms, while others have suggested that the oncogenic viruses must be introduced from outside as infectious agents for the causation of cancer. According to the viral oncogene hypothesis, chemical carcinogens, irradiation, and the normal aging process, all favour the partial or complete activation of viral oncogenes, possibly through gene mutations. On the other hand, following infection with an exogenous virus, the genotype of the infected cell is apparently altered, possibly due to partial or complete integration of the viral oncogene at certain site(s) in the cellular DNA, to give rise to a transformed cell. Although certain RNA and DNA viruses have been found to be associated with certain human malignancies, such as leukaemia (retroviruses), Burkitt's lymphoma, and cancers of the cervix and genital organs (herpes viruses), their precise role in the causation of human cancer remains unsettled. Tumour viruses may transform cells through several mechanisms. Some viruses may transform cells by insertion of their transforming genes into host cells, whose regulatory genes do not suppress the oncogene action. Other viruses might bring in some information that might act as a carcinogen affecting the regulatory components of the cell, and may cause cancer by directly impairing *R*-genes, or indirectly, by causing chromosome breaks at specific locations due to attachment at specific sites on certain chromosomes, which might lead to altered regulation due to deletion and/or position effect of tissue-specific *R*-genes.

A UNIFIED GENETIC CONCEPT OF CANCER

There has been a lot of discussion whether cancer originates as a consequence of mutational changes or developmental changes. This distinction is important since it has a bearing on the fact whether cancer is an irreversible or reversible process. If cancer arises following mutational events, then the cancerous process would very likely be irreversible. On the other hand, if cancer is due to developmental changes, then it would be potentially reversible. Spontaneous regressions of tumours to the normal state have been recorded. However, these are rather rare events. Although regression of tumours might be due to immunological mechanisms, those cases of reversal need to be fully examined, since reversal may not necessarily mean reversal to a completely 'normal state'. The revertant cells may still retain some of the properties of the progenitor cancer cells and often may represent a shift from the malignant to the benign tumour state. Based on these observations, I suggest that tumours may involve both mutational and developmental changes: That genetic and epigenetic theories of carcinogenesis are not mutually exclusive, but complementary if we consider tumour formation in the framework of a two-phase model of carcinogenesis consisting of *initiation* and *development* (Fig. 13.1). Each phase may further consist of two or more steps. The initiation phase may require up to two, or at the most, a few genetic changes (gene mutations,chromosome loss or rearrangements); this phase is probably irreversible. The developmental phase may involve two or more genetic and/ or epigenetic changes. If it consists of epigenetic changes, then the developmental phase is potentially reversible. In this model, the sites of genetic or epigenetic changes are regulatory genes (*R*-genes) that are specific for a given tissue or cell type. Changes in some of the putative *R* genes are involved in *initiation* (R_I genes); impairment of R_I gene(s), among other things, may result in decreased regulation of initiation of DNA synthesis. While changes in another set of *R* genes may be involved in the development (R_D genes) of neoplasia, impairment or a change of state of the R_D elements may result in aberrant cell differentiation. The expression of the malignant state may require a sequential and cumulative effect of genetic and epigenetic events involved in the initiation and developmental phases of carcinogenesis. In other words, the total cancer experience is a multistep process, presumably involving a genetic change in the R_I genes for the initiation phase, and an impairment or a change of state of R_D elements for the development and malignant expression. In the framework of this model, spontaneous or induced regression or reversal of tumour cells to the normal state may be centred on the developmental phase of carcinogenesis.

The initial genetic change probably results in a highly variable population of cells from which combinations advantageous to the expression and development of tumours may be selected. The malignant growth may result either from the loss of density-dependent regulation of growth, or from interaction of foetal gene derepressors with the genome to produce messenger RNA for the protein products involved in growth, invasiveness and metastasis. The two-phase genetic concept of carcinogenesis is compatible with the view – based on observations on somatic hybridization between malignant and normal cells in mouse and humans, and their subsequent inoculation in appropriate animal hosts – that different sets of genes are involved in the transformation (initiation) and malignant (developmental) phenotype. In other words, there is an apparent separation in the genetic control of initiation and development phases of carcinogenesis. The two-phase genetic concept of carcinogenesis is somewhat similar to the classical two-stage initiation and promotion model derived from the mouse skin carcinogenesis system. However, in the two-phase genetic concept, the genetic elements and the kind of changes involved in these elements in each phase are indicated.

In its simplest form, the two-phase model of carcinogenesis may involve genetic changes in two genes at a particular locus for initiation, followed by a few genetic and/or epigenetic changes at other loci to give rise to a cancerous cell. This kind of situation may be representative of human cancers whose predisposition is controlled in inheritance by one or two genes; for example, retinoblastoma and xeroderma pigmentosum. However, most human cancers, involving the lung, stomach, colon, and breast, probably require changes at more than two genes (very likely four to six mutations) for initiation and development of these cancers. It has been observed that initiation results from a limited dose of a carcinogen and is irreversible. On the other hand, development seems to depend upon prolonged exposure to so-called promoters. Although the precise mechanism of initiation of human cancer is unknown, it may be assumed that radiation and chemical carcinogens play an important role. It is also not clear what causes the development of cancer, but, as already pointed out, certain environmental factors appear to be good candidates; for example, tobacco

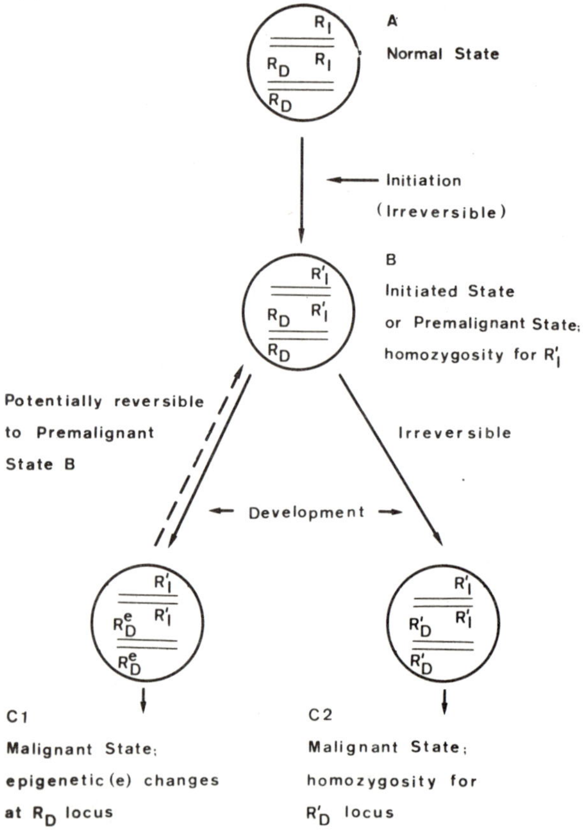

Fig. 13.1 **A two-phase genetic model of carcinogenesis. Diagram showing a normal cell (A) with two pairs of chromosomes (other chromosomes in the complement are not shown), carrying regulatory genes (*R*-genes), which prevent initiation (R_I) and development (R_D) of a neoplasm. Initiation (B) involves genetic changes**

(cont'd.)

smoke for lung cancer, and ingredients of diet (animal fat) for stomach and colon cancer. The promoters may be directly or indirectly involved in the development of cancer. However, in the absence of initiation, the promoters will not generally enhance the development phase of tumour formation. A number of agents have both initiating and promoting properties if given in sufficient doses over a period of time, and are called 'complete carcinogens'. Ingredients of tobacco smoke may have both initiating and promoting properties.

Following impairment or loss of regulatory or suppressor genes, the proto-*onc* genes may become active through several different mechanisms. One type of mechanism may involve amplification of the *onc* genes, that is, many more copies of the *onc* gene would be available. This results in overexpression of the oncogene. A second mechanism also relates to overexpression, but this may occur in a different way. The activity of the *onc* gene may be enhanced by the attachment of a strong transcriptional promoter element. The right promoter may turn a biologically inactive proto-oncogene into an overactive cancer gene. As a result of the foregoing mechanisms there would be enhanced production of gene products, i.e., the proteins, some of which are important in the initiation of tumourigenesis.

Thus, it would appear that two classes of genes may be involved in the origin of cancer: the tumour genes or

---

Fig. 13.1 *(cont'd.)* **(mutational events) in the R_I elements (represented by (R_I) and these changes are probably irreversible. The initiated cells may undergo differential growth to give rise to cancer (malignant growth) in one of the two different pathways involving changes in the R_1 elements and this mode of behaviour may, in part, be intrinsically determined by the cell type: when R_D genes undergo epigenetic changes (C1; represented by R_e) then the developmental phase is potentially reversible; on the other hand, when R_D elements involve genetic changes (mutations) (C2 represented by R_D) then the developmental phase would be irreversible.**

oncogenes and the regulatory genes or tumour suppressor genes (anti-oncogenes). Loss or mutation of an oncogene may lead to the loss of tumour formation ability in a specific tissue, whereas loss or mutation of a tumour suppressor gene would be oncogenic. The active role played by the oncogenes is apparent in certain leukaemias, lymphomas, and sarcomas, where specific chromosomal translocations have been observed. On the other hand, mutations in the second class of genes, the tumour suppressor genes, are more common in a broad spectrum of tumours, suggesting their primary involvement in the origin of cancer.

14

Experimental Systems in Cancer Research

In almost all forms of multicellular organisms, cancer is a disease in which living cells have lost the 'code of ethics' for normal behaviour and restraint and are, therefore, capable of aggressive expression. Cancer strikes, with equally devastating force, human beings as well as animals (monkeys, cows, dogs, cats, chickens, rats, mice, fish, and frogs, to mention some) and plants (tobacco, tomato, and many others). Extensive studies have been carried out on a number of plant and animal systems for the experimental production of tumours in order to discover the causes and mechanisms involved in the origin of cancer. These investigations have indicated that cancer can be induced by a multiplicity of diverse causes: for example, genetic imbalance or inheritance of certain defective genes; certain chemicals; radiations; and certain bacteria and viruses. However, the precise mechanisms of transformation from a normal to a cancer cell largely remain unknown. Some of the experimental systems in cancer research are discussed as follows.

THE CROWN GALL SYSTEM

By the turn of the twentieth century it was discovered that a specific bacterium was responsible for the initiation of tumour formation that is commonly known as *crown gall* disease in plants. Subsequently, the crown gall system has been extensively investigated in a number of different plant species, and has led to some understanding of the events in tumourigenesis. It is now known that for the initiation phase of tumourigenesis, a wound in a plant and a specific strain of bacteria, namely, *Agrobacterium tumefaciens*, are required. However, for the subsequent development of tumours, in the development phase, the bacterial presence is no longer necessary. During the developmental phase of tumourigenesis, certain growth-promoting substances, such as hormones, play an essential role in tumour formation. It seems that transformation of the normal cell into a tumour cell in crown gall disease involves progressive activation of certain biosynthetic systems, and the transformed cells so obtained become autonomous with respect to certain growth-promoting substances, particularly hormones, such as auxin and cytokinins. By growth autonomy it is implied that, following transformation, the tumour cells are capable of continuously synthesizing their hormones for cell reproduction and growth of tumours. In other words, gene systems involved in the synthesis of growth-promoting substances remain continuously active in the tumour cells, this activation being caused by the crown gall bacteria. On the other hand, the synthesis of the same growth-promoting substances, particularly the hormones, remains under stringent genetic control in the normal untransformed cells.

The crown gall bacteria carry a plasmid, the Ti (tumour-inducing) plasmid. It seems that the presence of the Ti plasmid is essential for the causation of the crown gall disease in plants. Several mutants have been discovered in the Ti plasmid that make it less tumourigenic or completely non-oncogenic. Plant cells (for example, tobacco) transformed by the disarmed (non-oncogenic) Ti plasmid can undergo normal growth and differentiation, and develop into normal plants. The Ti plasmid DNA was detected not only in these plants, but also in the progeny derived following reciprocal crosses between the transformed and the normal plants. This would indicate the transferred DNA (T-DNA) from the Ti plasmid was inherited through both female and male gametes as an integral plant gene. More recently, plasmid vector systems have been developed by recombinant DNA technology for genetic engineering and transfer of desirable genes into plants.

THE GENETIC TUMOUR SYSTEM IN TOBACCO

Another plant tumour system that has been extensively studied for over half a century is the tobacco (*Nicotiana*) genetic tumour system. For example, when two specific species of tobacco that are non-tumourous are crossed, the resulting hybrid plants develop normally until maturity (flowering stage) and then tumour formation occurs spontaneously on these plants (Fig. 14.1). Stresses of diverse nature, such as wounds, hormone treatments, chemicals, X-irradiation, and crowding seem to hasten the onset of tumours on these hybrid plants. All attempts to isolate a causative agent such as bacteria or viruses have failed. These observations suggest that the cancerous growths in the tobacco hybrids are genetically conditioned and require a non-specific stimulus to elicit tumour formation.

A large number of crosses have been made between different species of *Nicotiana* and all the hybrid combinations are not susceptible to tumour formation, but only certain hybrids develop tumours. This would indicate that certain genetic constellations, produced following hybridity, are more prone to cancer development than others. The tobacco species entering tumourous combinations have been divided

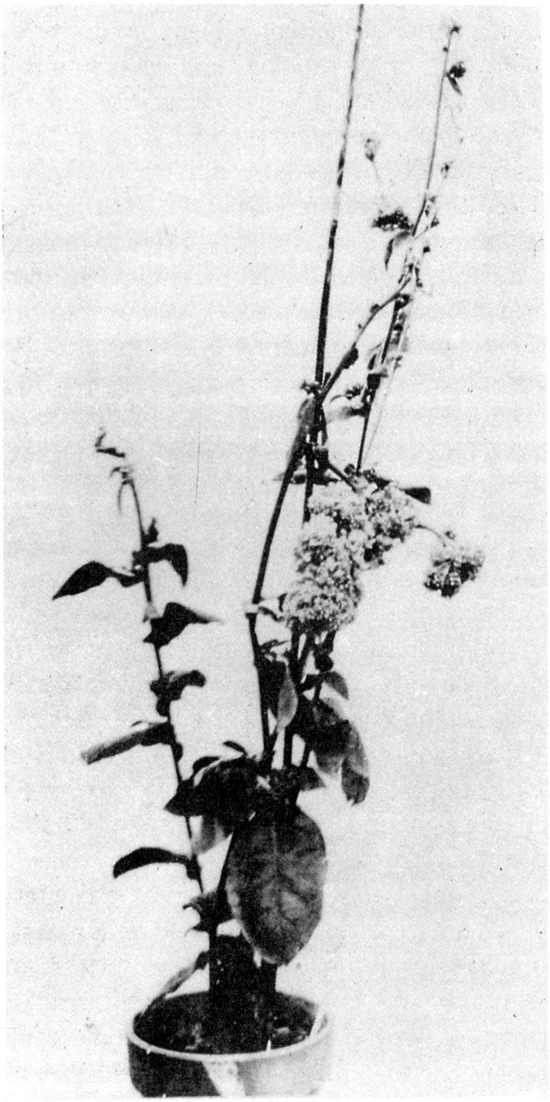

Fig. 14.1 Genetic tumours on a tobacco hybrid. The tumour trait is inherited from one generation to the next. The parental strains involved in such hybrids are entirely non-tumourous.

into two groups: one arbitrarily called the 'plus' group and the other the 'minus' group. Hybrids between a plus species and a minus species are tumourous, while hybrids within minus species only, or within the plus group only, are non-tumourous. From these studies it was concluded that critical contribution of the plus species to tumour formation in the hybrid must differ from that of the minus parent.

By appropriate crosses between the plus species and the minus species, it is possible not only to produce tumours at will but also to modify tumour expression to the extent that it is completely abolished. Detailed genetic analyses of two different hybrid combinations by further hybridizations (backcross analyses) have revealed that the two complementary genetic systems contributed by the plus species and the minus species in the hybrid are quite different. A single gene or a block of closely linked genes located on a specific chromosome seems to be an essential contribution by the plus species, whereas a number of genes distributed over many chromosomes of the minus species are required for tumour formation. Based on these observations, I have proposed a working hypothesis that tumour formation in tobacco is controlled in inheritance and probably initiated by a genetic element *I* (initiator) from the plus species. This initiator requires an appropriate genetic background provided by the minus parent to be expressed at all and, once initiated, the tumour expression and development are presumably enhanced by the action of the genetic elements *ee* (expression) representing more than one locus contributed by the minus parent.

The experimental evidence on the tobacco system has revealed that tumour formation occurs on individuals of specific genotypes. The initiation and development phases of tumour formation seem to be under the control of separate genetic loci. Although hybridization was employed for revealing the genetic control of tumour formation in tobacco, hybridization is not always essential for eliciting tumour development. Tumours arise on individuals in other plant and animal species, which are not necessarily hybrids. The question arises, whether non-tumour plus and minus parents have the potential for tumour formation. According to the genetic concept of cancer, either species would carry putative oncogene(s). However, in the plus species and the minus species the proto-oncogene expression is differently controlled, and the oncogene from the plus species is released from repression when it is transferred into the genetic background of the minus species by backcross hybridization. On the other hand, the proto-oncogene from the minus parent may be stringently controlled by a few *R* genes, perhaps requiring several mutational events. Consequently, in such cases, hybridization and mutagenesis may be required for releasing the proto-oncogene from suppression and initiation of tumourigenesis.

THE PLATYFISH-SWORDTAIL SYSTEM

A situation similar to that of genetic tumours in tobacco was discovered in the late 1920s in certain tropical fishes. Platyfish (*Xiphophorus maculatus*) and swordtail (*Xiphophorus helleri*) are found in rivers, brooks, and ponds in Mexico and adjacent areas in Central America. These fishes have been bred in captivity in aquaria for a long time, and, subsequently, pure bred strains of platyfish and swordtails and their hybrids have been investigated for gaining an understanding of the genetic basis of tumour formation, particularly melanoma formation and, in general, have led to ideas on the origin of cancer.

There are distinct spot-specific pigment cell (melanophores) patterns on the dorsal fin and skin of the platyfish strains, and each pattern is controlled in inheritance by a specific genetic locus. At least five spot-specific pigment cell patterns have been investigated in relation to melanoma formation in the platyfish-swordtail hybrids. However, only two sex-linked spot-specific loci from platyfish will be discussed here, namely, *Sd* (spotted black pattern on the dorsal fin) located on the X chromosome and *Sr* (striped pigment cell pattern on the bodyside) located on the Y chromosome. For example, when platyfish with the *Sd* pattern is crossed with a swordtail (which lacks the pigment cell pattern on the dorsal fin), the resulting F1 hybrids exhibit an enhanced expression of the pigment cells on the dorsal fin so that the entire dorsal fin becomes completely black, as compared to one or two black spots on the dorsal fin of pure bred platyfish (Fig. 14.2). This condition in the F1 hybrid results from somewhat abnormal proliferation/differentiation of the pigment cells and has been referred to as the *benign* melanoma condition. When such an F1 hybrid with benign melanoma is backcrossed to the swordtail, 25 per cent of the resulting offspring from this mating develop *malignant* melanoma, which may spread from the dorsal fin to the bodyside and may kill the fish; another 25 per cent of the progeny develop benign melanomas similar to those in the F1 hybrid, and the ramaining 50 per cent of the fishes are normal and resemble the swordtails (Fig. 14.2).

What is the explanation for these results? If we put both the malignant and benign melanoma-bearing fishes in one group, then there are 50 per cent animals with melanomas and the remaining 50 per cent without melanomas – the normal animals. This would represent a straightforward case of segregation at a locus in a heterozygous state (*Sd*/-) in a testcross. However, this further segregation of melanoma-bearing fish into malignant and benign groups requires a slightly different explanation and interpretation. There is substantial evidence to support the observation that in the platyfish the expression of the *Sd* pattern is stringently controlled, since deviations from the normal *Sd* pattern have not been observed in the natural tropical habitat or under the aquaria conditions in the platyfish. This regulation of the *Sd* locus in platyfish seems to be accomplished mainly by a

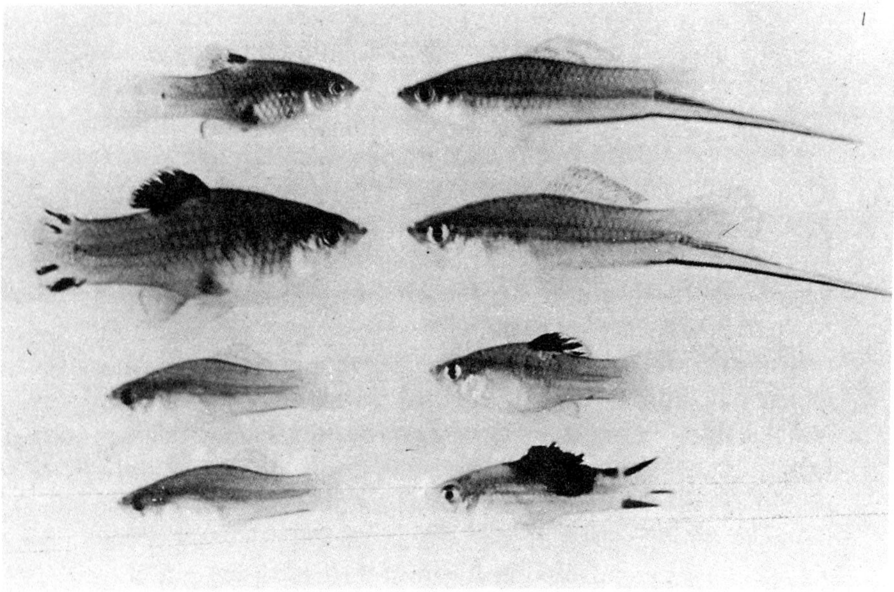

Fig. 14.2 Melanoma formation in the platyfish and swordtail hybrids. The parental strains (top row) are normal; platyfish (top left) has two pigmented spots (*Sd*) on the dorsal fin. When a platyfish is crossed to a swordtail (top right), the F1 hybrids (second row left) develop benign melanomas on the dorsal fin. Crossing the F1 to swordtail (second row right) yields progeny, 50 per cent of which develop melanomas (25 per cent benign and 25 per cent malignant) as shown in the bottom two rows (right), and 50 per cent of the fishes are melanoma-free (bottom two rows, left). The melanomas in these fishes are genetically conditioned by the tumour genes (Tu) and are inherited. (*Courtesy*: Professor Fritz Anders, Giessen, Germany.)

pair of regulatory genes (*R* genes). As it turns out, the regulatory genes that control the expression of the *Sd* pattern are not located on the X chromosomes on which *Sd* is located, but on different chromosomes. Since the swordtail fish has no pigment spot pattern on the dorsal fin, it is reasonable to assume that it has no regulatory genes for the control of the pigment cell pattern. The crossing of platyfish with the genotype *Sd/Sd, R/R* to a swordtail with genetic constitution -/-, -/- (lacking both loci) yields F1 progeny with the genotype *Sd/-, R/-* and these animals develop benign melanomas because of the loss of the one *R* gene due to mating, which results in less controlled regulation of pigment cell reproduction/differentiation in the dorsal fin area and consequently leads to benign melanomas. By further crossing the F1 hybrid (*Sd/-, R/-*) with benign melanoma to swordtail (-/-, -/-), an independent assortment of *Sd/* - and *R/-* loci results in the folllowing three classes: Class I (25 per cent) carrying *Sd/-*, -/- (lacking the specific *R* gene from platyfish) in the swordtail genome develop malignant melanomas because of poorly controlled pigment cell reproduction and differentiation due to loss of the *R* genes; Class II (25 per cent) fishes have the genetic constitution *Sd/-, R/-*, and develop benign melanomas; Class III (50 per cent) fishes which lack both *Sd* and *R* genes (-/-, -/-), therefore do not develop melanomas on the dorsal fin. The genetic scheme for the *Sd*-conditioned melanoma development is shown in Fig. 14.2.

Another pigment cell spotting pattern determining gene *Sr* is located on the Y chromosome of the platyfish. Under normal conditions *Sr* determines the striped expression of the flank above the midlateral line and in front of the dorsal fin of the platyfish. When the platyfish with the *Sr* pattern is mated to the swordtail (which has neither *Sr* pattern on its bodyside nor its controlling genes), the resulting F1 hybrid offspring do not develop benign melanomas on the bodyside, but the *Sr* pattern in these hybrid fishes remains rather similar to that in the pure bred platyfish. Even when the *Sr*-carrying F1 hybrid is further backcrossed to the swordtail, no melanomas develop on the bodyside of the resulting fishes. On the other hand, when pure-bred platyfish with the *Sr* pattern or hybrids between the *Sr* platyfish and the swordtail is irradiated with X-rays, a very small proportion of fishes develop melanomas on the bodyside.

What is the explanation for such a result? As in the case of *Sd*, the *Sr* pattern is strictly regulated on the bodyside of the fish. Contrasted to the *Sd* pattern, which is controlled by regulatory genes that are located on different chromosomes from the *Sd* itself (this is known as *unlinked* or *non-linked* conditions of genes), the *Sr* and its regulatory gene are both located on the same *Y* chromosome. The *Sr* and its main *R* gene must be very closely linked since no tumourous recombinants were recovered in the hybrid offspring. Melanoma developed on the irradiated *Sr* platyfish or its hybrids with the swordtail, presumably due to a genetic change (mutational event) in the *R* gene.

Since *Sd* and *Sr* are involved in melanoma or tumour formation, they have been called *Tu* (tumour) genes, and their controlling genes have been designated as regulatory genes (*R* genes). Impairment of the *R* gene function or deletion of *R* genes due to mutational events, or loss of *R* genes due to selective matings, results in the activation of *Tu* genes, which leads to loss of control over cell reproduction and cell differentiation in the target cells; in this case, pigment cells. In a certain stock of the platyfish where the *Sd* pattern was lost due to a mutation in the *Sd* locus, the fishes also lost the ability to develop melanomas on the dorsal fin of the hybrids between the *Sd* deletion platyfish and swordtails. Chromosomal studies on the *Sd* platyfish stock revealed that *Sd* (*Tu*) locus is located in a terminal region of the X chromosome, and in the *Sd* deletion stock there was a corresponding loss of the terminal segment of the X chromosome, thus providing credence to the presence of inherent tumour-inducing genetic information in the cells of fish.

The foregoing investigations on the platyfish-swordtail melanoma system suggest that impairment or loss of *R* genes, on the one hand, presumably leads to neoplastic development, whereas loss or impairment of *Tu* genes, on the other hand, would lead to loss of tumour-forming potential in specific tissues. And loss of *Tu* genes might represent a potential mechanism involved in reversal from tumour to the normal state.

THE MOUSE SYSTEM

Around 1915 it was discovered that repeated applications of tar to the ears of rabbits produced skin cancer. Very soon thereafter, the same experimental procedure also produced skin cancer in mice. Subsequently, various inbred lines of mice became available that had been selected for spontaneously occurring high and low incidence of different cancers, and in particular leukaemia or mammary cancer. The availability of such lines made the mouse the most convenient animal for experimental cancer research.

Mammary Cancer

Extensive studies have been carried out on the factors that influence the production of mammary or breast cancer in mice. These investigations have revealed that development of mammary cancer in mice is probably determined by three factors: (1) an inherited mammary cancer predisposition, (2) the Bittner milk virus, and (3) a hormonal influence. For example, when high- and low-incidence mammary cancer strains in mice are mated, the incidence of mammary tumours in the F1 hybrid females depends on whether they are foster-nursed by mothers with a high- or low-incidence strain. Many mammary tumours developed when the F1 females were foster-nursed by mothers with the high-incidence strain. On the other hand, those females foster-nursed on mothers from low-incidence mammary cancer strain developed very few mammary tumours. These studies indicated that there was some kind of transmission of an agent or factor through the milk in the high-incidence mammary cancer strains from the mothers to the daughters. The causative agent in mice was found to be a virus, the Bittner virus (named after the discoverer), transmitted through the milk. Such a mechanism of virus transmission does not seem to be important in human breast cancer. In many strains of mice genetic transmission (through the germline) of mouse mammary tumour virus (MMTV), occurs, and variation in tumour incidence seems to be associated with variability in genetic expression of MMTV. In humans, genetic predisposition and alteration in the female hormone seem to determine the breast cancer risk.

Leukaemia

There is considerable experimental evidence to demonstrate that certain viruses cause leukaemias in a variety of animals, including mice. Many laboratory strains of mice harbour leukaemia viruses (retroviruses) in their tissues, which may remain dormant, without necessarily causing the disease. Leukaemia viruses may be inherited in certain strains of mice through the germline, while, in others, the virus may be spread horizontally (as an infection). When present in the dormant form, the leukaemia virus may be activated by a variety of different environmental factors. Leukaemia viruses have often been found in leukaemic cells in mice where the disease has been brought about by chemical agents, radiation, or even diet. Some inbred strains of mice exhibit a high incidence of leukaemia associated with massive production of a virus called MLV (murine leukaemia virus) when the animals are about six months' old. The murine leukaemia incidence can, however, be greatly reduced or prevented by greatly restricting the diet. On the other hand, well-fed mice under the laboratory conditions show a high incidence of murine leukaemia. It has been suggested that this disease may be triggered off initially by slight imbalance between virus production and immune response, and this imbalance, among other things, may be caused by restricting the diet.

Do leukaemia viruses occur naturally in other mammals, including humans? Here, mention may be made of a human pet, the cat, which harbours a leukaemia virus, FeLV (feline leukaemia virus). This virus spreads horizontally, that is, from one cat to another as an infectious agent and is the major cause of leukaemia and lymphosarcomas in the cat. Most infected cats develop strong antibody response and become immune to FeLV. But, occasionally, something seems to go wrong with the immune response, and the cat can suffer either a massive destruction of the immune system, or continued uncontrolled proliferation of the lymphocytes, and the virus leads to the onset of leukaemia or lymphosarcoma. Although the leukaemia viruses have not been found to occur naturally in humans, footprints of leukaemia retroviruses have been detected in the blood cells from many leukaemic patients.

Teratocarcinoma

Teratocarcinoma is a malignant tumour of embryonal origin in the mouse. This tumour occurs rather rarely in this mammal. Typically, teratocarcinoma consists of two major components: an undifferentiated cell component and the differentiated constituent. The undifferentiated mass forms the embryonal carcinoma cells, representing the malignant constituent of the tumour. These tumour cells are dispersed among a variety of differentiated cell types, ranging from 8 to 14, including epithelial cells, nerve cells, muscle, bone and cartilage cells, tooth buds and hair follicles. Upon transplantation of such a tumour from one mouse to another a broad spectrum of cell types, typical of teratocarcinoma, are reproduced indefinitely. Questions arose as to the origin of the differentiated cell in the tumour: whether such cell types develop independently? Or did they all arise from a common precursor or stem cell? In this context, teratocarcinoma has not only served as a model system for testing whether carcinoma cells are developmentally totipotent, that is, they have a potential to give rise to differentiated cell types, but also for testing the hypothesis whether cancer arises epigenetically, that is, due to a change in the developmental process, and if so, then cancer is potentially reversible.

In order to test the totipotency of the tumour cells, single embryonal carcinoma cells were injected into the peritonial cavities of mice. In about half the instances, the single cells established themselves and grew into malignant tumours that killed the animals. Histological examination of the tumours revealed that they were composed of a chaotic array of 8 to 14 differentiated cell types along with the undifferentiated embryonal carcinoma cells, characteristic of a teratocarcinoma.

To further test the totipotency of tumour cells in the environment of a normal mouse embryo, and to ascertain whether cancer is reversible, the embryonal carcinoma cells carrying specific markers, for example, specific liver proteins, melanin, and certain other enzyme markers in blood, were injected into blastocytes (early embryos) of a strain of mouse lacking these genetic markers by Beatrice Mintz and her associates. The mice that developed from the injected embryos were free of teratocarcinoma, but showed the genetic markers of the embryonal carcinoma cells. This study indicates that tumour-derived cells had contributed significantly to the development of normal tissues (as monitored by genetic markers) and remained developmentally totipotent in an appropriate environment and failed to form any tumour cells. Taken together, these experiments with the mouse teratocarcinoma system have been interpreted to imply that transformation from a normal state to a malignant state and reversal to normalcy result from a change in gene expression (developmental or epigenetic change) rather than in gene structure (mutational event). The observations in mouse teratocarcinoma may also be explained in other ways. For example, a normal differentiating cell may be recovered in which malignant properties are suppressed following the fusion of carcinoma and normal cells in the embryo. Alternatively, the original transforming mutation may be unstable in an environment in the early mouse embryo that specifically promotes the differentiation of normal cells. In other words, the genes in the normal embryo may abolish or suppress the carcinogenic properties of the carcinoma cells.

THE HUMAN SYSTEM

Although human beings cannot be used for experimental production of cancer, we have gained a lot of insight into the cancer problem from studies on spontaneously occurring tumours in the following categories: (a) inherited predisposition to certain cancers; (b) specific chromosome syndromes associated with certain cancers; and (c) strong association between environmental factors and cancers of specific organ sites in the human population. The observations on human cancers from these three categories (discussed in detail in several chapters of this book) have led to the general hypothesis that genetic change, resulting from gene-environment interaction, seems to be the underlying cause for the origin of cancer. This conclusion has been considerably strengthened from investigations on animal and plant tumour systems. All the different types of cancers occurring in humans have been experimentally produced in animals by genetic manipulations, or exposure to certain environmental factors, for example, chemical, carcinogens, and in many cases the tumours are at the same site and of the same biological type as the human tumours.

NORMAL CELLS AND CANCER CELLS *IN VITRO*

In order to compare the properties of normal cells and cancer cells, attempts have been made to culture cells in vessels or tubes from a variety of different organisms, including mammals: for example, mouse, rat, hamster, monkey, and humans. Another objective of the cell culture research has been to study the process of *transformation*, that is, conversion of a normal cell into a cancer cell. Although normal and cancer cells have been investigated *in vitro* (in a culture vessel) in several plants and animals, we shall briefly mention here some of the salient points from the mammalian cell research.

Differences between Normal and Cancer Cells

When normal cells are grown on a nutrient medium, the cells can proliferate for several months under the culture conditions, and, if they remain normal, they eventually cease to divide and die. The cancer cells, on the other hand, continue to proliferate for years under culture conditions, without showing any loss of viability. In fact, one of the first human cells to be cultured successfully, which also happens to be a cancer cell line, was derived in 1951 from the cancer cells of an African-American woman Henrieta Lack, who died of cervical cancer. However, her cancerous cells dubbed *HeLa* (named after the first two letters of her two names) have achieved immortality.

When normal and cancer cells, after having been in culture for a long duration of time, are implanted into the normal test animals, it is noted that the normal cells cease to proliferate and the animal is not harmed in any way, whereas reimplanted cancer cells continue to multiply and eventually kill the test animal.

Another very interesting and puzzling difference is the way normal and cancer cells behave when they become crowded in culture. Normal cells, *in vitro*, continue to multiply in the glass container till the surface is completely covered by cells. But the moment the normal cells become crowded, they seem to automatically stop reproduction of new cells. The cancer cells in culture, on the other hand, behave quite differently. They seem to lack the built-in control mechanism for the inhibition of cell reproduction when crowding occurs. The cancer cells continue to multiply in spite of close contact and start piling haphazardly on top of one another thus forming masses of cancer cells. In other words, the cancer cells lack contact inhibition, which is characteristic of normal cells.

Thus, cancer cells grown in culture behave in a similar manner as they do in the organism. They proliferate continuously without any restraint, spreading in all directions – like an uncontrollable flood destroying everything that is normal. Why does a cancer cell behave differently from a normal cell? What is the built-in control mechanism in the normal cell that restrains it from abnormal proliferation? These are some of the basic questions that need to be investigated at the biochemical and molecular levels for a better understanding of normal and abnormal cell reproduction and differentiation.

Transformation

When small pieces of mouse tissue are placed in a culture vessel containing a nutrient medium, the cells which grow the best are the *fibroblasts*, named thus because of their appearance. The cells reproduce and eventually may cover the entire floor of the culture vessel. At this stage the fibroblasts can be detached by treating them with the proteolytic enzyme trypsin, and some of the detached cells can be seeded in fresh vessels containing a nutrient medium, where they can settle down and start multiplying again. By this procedure normal cells can be kept alive for several months, but eventually the cells cease to reproduce and die. Sometimes, however, variants that have a different style of growth behaviour can arise in the cell culture. Instead of spreading flat on the floor of the culture vessel like the normal fibroblasts, the variant cells are piled one upon another. This change, which is called transformation, imparts a selective advantage to the transformed cells so obtained, which proliferate continuously to dominate the culture. When cells that have undergone transformation in the culture are reimplanted in the mice, they often form tumours.

Transformation can be induced in cultured normal cells by certain chemicals, viruses, and radiation that are known to cause cancer in animals. Transformed cells so obtained tend to be tumourigenic in experimental animals. Therefore, transformation in cultured cells offers opportunities for analysing the initial events of carcinogenesis under controlled conditions, and finding out what exactly the various carcinogenic agents are doing to the cellular machinery.

Transformation occurs at varied frequencies in cultured cells from different animals. For example, the appearance of spontaneously transformed variants is fairly common in cultured mouse cells; it is rather infrequent in rat and hamster cells, and virtually unknown in human cells. Cells that undergo spontaneous transformation can be transformed into tumourigenic cells fairly efficiently by chemical carcinogens, viruses and radiation. Human cells, which hardly undergo spontaneous transformation *in vitro*, can be transformed by viruses, but rather infrequently by chemical carcinogens and radiation. The mouse cells, on the other hand, are readily transformed by chemical carcinogens and radiation. We do not know what protects human cells from becoming transformed *in vitro* following exposure to chemical or physical mutagens. Several possibilities present themselves. The differential frequencies of transformation in human and mouse cells may be due to: (a) the way the constellation of genes is organized for the prevention of transformation (the human cells may have relatively more controlling genes than mouse cells); (b) the difference in the susceptibility may be related to the life span of humans (long-lived) and mouse (short-lived); and (c) the culture conditions under which the cells are kept alive, which are far removed from conditions in the living organism. Therefore, great caution should be exercised while extrapolating transformation results obtained from mouse cells maintained in culture vessels to the human cancer problem.

15

Detection of Cancer

The early detection of cancer poses one of the most challenging problems in cancer research. A good deal of scientific effort is directed towards discovering early warning signals with respect to cancer. Since most human cancers seem to have a relatively long 'latent period' ranging anywhere from 5 to 20 years before they develop, the cancer symptoms, therefore, are not well defined in the early spectrum of the 'latent period'. This problem is even more complicated in the cancer of internal tissues or organs, where hundreds of millions of cancer cells are produced even before the detection of the early stages of the disease. The longer the cancer of the internal tissues remains undetected, the greater the likelihood that migration of cancer cells to other parts of the body has occurred, leading to the establishment of new cancerous colonies. At that stage it becomes extremely difficult to control the disease. Therefore, the early detection of cancer minimizes the probability of metastasis and increases the effectiveness of the treatment. Unfortunately, more than half of all cancers develop life-threatening metastases (that is, spread to other parts of the body) before they are finally detected with the help of modern techniques. If tumours could be detected during the early stages of development, while they are still very small and localized, the cure rates could be as high as 90 per cent, as compared to the 40 per cent that are now controlled.

CANCER WARNING SIGNALS

There are several warning signals which indicate that cancer may be present. However, these signals may not necessarily mean that an individual is afflicted by cancer. Nevertheless, they should not be ignored, if they persist over a couple of weeks. The American Cancer Society has listed the following warning symptoms:

- Change in bowel or bladder habits.
- A sore that does not heal.
- Unusual bleeding or discharge.
- Thickening or lump in the breast or elsewhere.
- Indigestion or difficulty in swallowing.
- Obvious change in a wart or mole.
- Nagging cough or hoarseness.

These symptoms can be caused by cancer or by a number of other medical problems. They should be taken seriously. If they persist, consult a doctor.

BIOCHEMICAL MARKERS FOR EARLY DETECTION OF CANCER

A large number of investigators have been searching for biochemical markers that reveal the presence of cancer long before the clinical symptoms become apparent. Like the relatively simple *pap smear* test routinely used for detecting cervical cancer, the biochemical tests are also simple so that they can be easily performed on individuals at a high risk of cancer or for screening the general population. The biochemical markers indicative of the presence of cancer have, in recent years, been mostly investigated in the blood and, to a limited extent, in the urine. Some of the biochemical markers were considered to be specific for certain cancers, but subsequent investigations revealed these tests to be non-specific. Nevertheless, the use of biochemical markers offers a promising approach for the early detection of cancer as well as for monitoring the course of cancer therapy. Several biochemical markers are based on preliminary experiments, and therefore would require further confirmation with regard to their association with cancer.

MARKERS IN BLOOD

Carcinoembryonic Antigen (CEA)

Earlier studies indicated elevated levels of CEA to be a specific marker for cancer of the colon. However, subsequent studies by a large number of investigators have shown that elevated levels of CEA also appear in the blood of patients with many other types of tumours, and in individuals who smoke heavily or in individuals with certain non-malignant conditions. For these reasons CEA does not represent a practical screening method for cancer. But preliminary results suggest that CEA has a great value for monitoring the course of cancer therapy: CEA levels in blood decline if cancer therapy produces regression, and rise again if there is a recurrence of the disease. For example, rising levels of CEA have been used to predict a recurrence of the tumours of colon, breast and rectum with a high probability (above 70 per cent), and the gradual rise in CEA levels generally occurred 9 to 12 months before the clinical symptoms of the disease became apparent.

Alfa Fetoprotein (AFP)

High concentrations of AFP have been found in the blood of individuals with liver cancer and certain other cancers. Like CEA, the AFP has also been used in monitoring the cancer therapy.

AFP and CEA are the prototypes of the so-called oncofoetal antigens that are present in foetal tissues but are normally not present or, when present, only in very small amounts in healthy adult tissues.

Prostate Acid Phosphatase (PAP)

Higher levels of PAP have been detected in the blood of patients with prostate cancer. By employing this method about 50 per cent of the localized prostate tumours and about 80 per cent of the more advanced cases have been detected. In addition, levels of another protein, prostate-specific antigen (PSA) may also rise in those who have prostate cancer or benign prostatic hypertrophy. These biochemical markers appear to be specific for detecting prostrate tumours and are now routinely employed in screening individuals at a high risk of prostate cancer.

Glycoproteins

A glycoprotein has been found to be specifically associated with breast tumours, and it is also present in human breast cancer cells maintained in tissue culture. Another glycoprotein has been observed so far only in tumours of the pancreas. Attempts are being made to devise sensitive enough methods to detect these glycoproteins in the blood of patients facing a high risk of cancer of the breast and pancreas.

B-Protein

Abnormal levels of B-protein are present in the blood of patients with more than one type of tumour; for example, tumours of the breast, skin, and internal organs. B-protein has also been found to be associated with non-malignant conditions.

C3DP

This is a protein that binds itself to DNA. It is present in much higher concentrations in the blood of patients with leukaemias, lymphomas, and melanomas than in healthy individuals. C3DP concentrations correlate with the severity of the malignancy, and in a majority of cases it is a useful marker for monitoring therapy.

Carbohydrates

Sugars bound to proteins in the blood may serve as markers for cancer detection. It has been found that concentrations of sialic acid, hexoses, and fructoses are higher in cancer patients than in healthy individuals. The increased concentrations of these substances seem to be correlated with the severity of the disease.

Hormones

Human chorionic gonadotrophin (HCG), known as the pregnancy hormone, has been found to be associated with various malignancies. HCG is frequently used as one of the markers for monitoring therapy for choriocarcinoma and testicular tumours. High concentrations of the precursor of another hormone, adrenocorticotropic hormone (ACTH), have been found in many patients with lung cancer.

MARKERS IN URINE

Compared to the number of biochemical markers investigated in blood, the number searched for in urine has been limited. This is somewhat surprising because most patients with disseminated cancers have been found to excrete as much as a gram of protein through urine each day. By contrast, the healthy individuals excrete little or no protein. Five proteins have been purified and it has been found that one or more of these proteins appear in the urine of about 70 per cent of the patients with disseminated cancers and in a smaller percentage of cases with localized tumours.

Another class of substances found in urine is *polyamines*. Changes in the concentrations of polyamines in urine are useful for monitoring chemotherapy in patients with Burkitt's lymphoma, melanomas, leukaemias and cancers of the colon, rectum and brain.

The aforementioned are some of the biochemical markers that seem to hold promise for the early detection of cancer. Although most of these markers are non-specific, that is, more than one cancer is associated with one marker, the use of multiple markers provides the best opportunities not only for early detection of cancer, but also for monitoring regression or recurrence of the disease during the course of therapy.

16

Strategies for the Control of Human Cancer

There are about 100 different types of human cancer. Although all cancers may share some common basic mechanism(s) for their origin, their expression depends on the cell type involved, and, therefore, each cancer has the attributes and the chemistry related to the cell type of its origin. Cancer of the skin is very different from the cancer of the lung or the cancer of white blood cells (leukaemia). Therefore, strategies for control of different forms of cancer have to be evolved that prolong the quality of life in each case. One of the major objectives of cancer research is to find out what causes the disease, so that this knowledge can be effectively utilized to control human cancer, which is one of the major causes of death. It seems unlikely that any single factor, genetic or environmental, alone causes cancer. The ultimate answer to what really causes cancer may lie in discovering the precise nature of genetic and environmental interactions that determine whether a cell will continue to be normal or would deviate to a cancerous pathway. Therefore, in order to learn more about the cancer cell, we must first have a better understanding of the genetics, molecular biology, biochemistry, and behaviour of normal cells, particularly in the area of control of cell reproduction and cell differentiation – the two processes at the heart of the very basis of life! We have come a long way in terms of our understanding of the basic processes of living cells, but still a great deal remains to be learned. And it may be quite a long while before we are able to fathom most of, but not all, the secrets of a living cell. When we accomplish that, we may be in a better position to minimize cancer risk. Meanwhile, we must continue our fight against cancer and find ways and means to control it.

TREATMENT OF CANCER

There are several different methods for the treatment or control of cancer. Surgery, radiation, and chemotherapy (drug treatment) are being widely employed by therapists to treat cancer. In addition, some interesting biological approaches to control cancer, based on differences between normal and tumour cells, are still in the experimental stages. Most promising results are obtained when cancer is detected at an early stage of development, that is, before the number of cancer cells has become too large and before the cancer cells have migrated to other parts of the body, and every cancer cell is removed and destroyed.

Surgery and Radiation

Surgery and radiation are the two major components of the strategy against localized forms of cancer. Surgery is the weapon most widely used for attack on tumours. Complete cure is achieved when every single cancer cell is removed by surgical means. Failures after surgery are largely due to the distant spread of cancer cells. Surgery is remarkably successful for certain kinds of tumours. It is the primary form of therapy responsible for extending survival for 5 years in 85 per cent of patients with skin cancer, in 70 per cent of women with breast cancer, and in about 40 per cent of patients with cancer of the colon.

Radiation is the secondmost powerful weapon in the hands of cancer therapists. It is particulary useful for treating internal solid tumours if they are detected at an early stage of development. When tumours are detected early, radiotherapy is responsible for extending survival for 5 years in 90 per cent of men with seminoma (one type of cancer of the testis), in at least 80 per cent of children with retinoblastoma (a cancer of the eye), in about 75 per cent of patients with Hodgkin's disease (a cancer of the lymph system), and in about 50 per cent of patients with cancer of the nasopharynx.

Destruction of cancer cells by radiation is based, in part, on the reproductive profile of the cancer cells. In general, dividing cells are more easily destroyed by radiation than non-dividing cells: the more frequently the cells divide, the more sensitive they are to radiation killing. Since cancer cells are constantly multiplying populations of cells, they are more susceptible to radiation damage than are normal non-dividing cells. However, not all the normal cells in our bodies are non-dividing. Normal cells also reproduce to replace worn out dead cells, depending upon the demands of replacement of cells in each tissue. For example, bone marrow cells multiply at a relatively higher rate to replace the dying circulating cells faster than most kinds of cancer cells, including cancer cells of the white blood cells, and, therefore, they are more sensitive to radiation damage than any other cancer cell. Cells lining the intestine also multiply frequently in order to replace their dead cells. The blood-forming cells and the dividing intestine cells are, therefore, highly prone to radiation damage. When a person is exposed to high levels of radiation, he or she develops radiation sickness mainly due to failure of these two tissues. It is ironical indeed that radiation therapy used for curing cancer in one organ may cause damage and destruction of normal dividing cells of another tissue, and may also cause cancer by inducing genetic change (mutations) in a third tissue. These are some of the problems associated with radiation therapy of cancer.

Both surgery and radiation therapy have their limitations in that they are generally useful only against localized tumours. Surgery by using laser beams offers a new kind of perspective in cancer therapy. Treatment with radiation is still improving by virtue of improvement in focussing the radiation dose on the tumour, and from exploitation of alternative forms of radiation such as fast neutrons. Surgery and radiation therapy are, however, ineffective against cancer that has undergone metastasis and has spread to distant sites in the body, which is the cause of at least half of all cancer deaths.

Chemotherapy

Chemotherapy is the primary form of treatment against several types of disseminated cancers. Anti-tumour drug treatment has been used with notable success against leukaemias and lymphomas such as Burkitt's lymphoma and Hodgkin's disease. In addition, chemotherapy has been frequently employed against cancers which have spread to distant locations after the primary tumour has been irradicated by surgery or radiation. This type of adjunct chemotherapy has been attempted with some success against several childhood malignancies.

Wilm's tumour is a lethal cancer of the kidney in children. Surgery or radiation therapy has produced a cure rate (2-year survival) in about 25 per cent of the patients. A combination of surgery and radiation treatments increases the cure rates to about 40 per cent. A combination of three treatments, namely, surgery and radiation therapy followed by the anti-tumour drug actinomycin D, increases the cure rate to more than 80 per cent. Embryonal rhabdomyosarcoma, a muscle tumour that generally develops after birth, exhibits the same responsiveness to surgery and radiation treatment as Wilm's tumour of the kidney. However, combined treatment with surgery, radiation, and anti-tumour drugs seems to produce long-term disease-free survival.

Chemotherapy has also been applied to cancers other than the spreading type, particularly small tumours that have developed recently. It is much less effective against tumours that are comparatively older and larger. The most important difference between young and old tumours is that the young tumour consists of a large fraction of actively dividing cells compared to a relatively small fraction of dividing cells in the older tumours. Since most anti-tumour drugs act by interfering with the cell cycle and selectively kill cells that are actively reproducing, the large fractions of growing cells in the young tumours makes them highly susceptible to the killing effects of anti-tumour drugs. By contrast, a small fraction of growing cells in the older tumours makes them less susceptible to chemotherapy. The selective destruction of cancer cells by anti-tumour drugs and radiation treatment presents the same kind of problems, as discussed in the previous section, as for actively dividing normal cells. Unfortunately, both these therapeutic agents indiscriminately destroy actively dividing cells, whether they are cancer cells or normal cells. Besides, most anti-tumour drugs have varied side-effects associated with their toxicity to healthy cells. Since the beginning of the chemotherapy programme in the early 1950s, many thousands of drugs have been tested, and only a small proportion of these are currently used to treat cancer. However, anti-tumour drugs that selectively kill cancer cells and are absolutely 'safe' for normal cells have yet to be discovered. These discoveries will ultimately depend upon pinpointing specific biochemical differences between normal cells and cancer cells, and then focussing the chemical attack on the most sensitive biochemical 'hot spots' of the cancer cells, but without damaging the normal cells.

Hyperthermia

Treatment of cancer with heat has always intrigued physicians. According to a 5000-year-old papyrus writing, the ancient Egyptians practised a 'fire drill', that is, a heated stick was inserted into tumours to treat them. Physicians in the last century observed that malignant tumours sometimes disappeared when patients developed high fever. Hyperthermia, that is, treatment of cancer with heat-generating microwaves and radiowaves, is developing into a promising new approach. Microwaves generate heat by causing rapid oscillation of water and protein molecules in the cells. Heat tends to remain in the tumour, which apparently has a poor blood circulation, and kills the tumour cells. On the other hand, heat is rapidly dissipated from the surrounding normal tissues by the flow of blood, and consequently may not harm the normal cells. By focussing the beams of microwaves or radiowaves on tumours, many doctors are currently treating patients with tumours of the brain, lung, liver, and other malignancies. In combination with chemotherapy and radiation treatment, hyperthermia seems to work best because heat apparently tends to render cancer cells more susceptible to chemical and radiation damage.

Immunological Control

Our bodies are protected against infections from bacteria or viruses by the immune system. The functions of the immune system are to recognize alien substances entering the body and to destroy them. The cells of the immune system recognize specific targets (antigens) of the alien cells or substances and eliminate them through antibodies or killer cells. Circulating antibodies or killer cells discriminate between the body's own substances and those foreign to the body.

Each type of substance (antigen) introduced into the body through an infectious bacterium or a virus invokes a specific immune response and stimulates the production of antibodies or specifically sensitized killer cells.

Cancer cells differ from normal cells in that a new antigen is present on the surface of the tumour cells. It is suspected that the tumour antigen may be recognized by the immune system as a foreign substance especially in early tumours, and the defence system may keep many early tumours in check. Spontaneous regression of advanced tumours has been also attributed to the immunological defence system. However, in general, the immune system fails to recognize the tumour antigen, and therefore does not attack and destroy the cancer cells. The reasons for the failure of the immune system to eliminate cancer cells are not well understood. A recent development in cancer therapy has been to modify the surface of the cancer cells in order to invoke an immune response. The immunoadjuvants commonly used are of non-specific types involving bacterial or fungal products. Following the injection of large quantities of some very powerful antigen, for example, an attenuated form of tubercle bacillus (tuberculosis), dramatic remissions have been reported for several types of cancers. The precise mechanisms by which these non-specific immunoadjuvants stimulate the immune response against cancer cells have not yet been understood.

Hormone Therapy

Some types of cancer require hormones for their growth. In such cases, control strategies may involve preventing the cancer cells from getting the hormone for their growth. One approach might include the use of drug(s) that block(s) the production of a specific hormone. Alternatively, the organ/ gland producing that hormone may be removed from the body by surgery. Hormone therapy has been frequently employed to treat cancers of the breast, prostate, kidney, and uterus. Drugs commonly used in hormone therapy include tamoxifen (for breast cancer), diethylstilbestrol or DES (for breast and prostate cancers), and Megace (for kidney and uterine cancers).

A number of side-effects may be caused by hormone therapy, depending on the specific anti-hormone drug or surgical procedure. These side-effects might include nausea and vomiting, swelling, or weight gain, and, in some cases, the treatment interferes with the body's production and use of hormones. For example, women taking tamoxifen against breast cancer may experience pseudo-menopause symptoms, such as hot flushes.

BIOLOGICAL THERAPY (IMMUNOTHERAPY)

Interferons

Interferons are small glycoprotein molecules that are released from cells infected with a virus. These substances diffuse to neighbouring cells and protect those cells not only from the virus initially involved in establishing infection but also from other kinds of viral infection. It is now believed that viral infections are generally held in check as a result of the interferon-mediated defence mechanism. Interferons have been found to have detectable effects in not only preventing the transformation process in certain virally initiated tumours, but also arresting progression as well as causing regression in certain advanced tumours in mice by selectively killing cancer cells. Although interferons are not toxic substances by themselves, even in moderately large doses, sometimes toxic symptoms develop in the treated animals due to sudden killing and massive lysis of cancer cells.

Studies with the use of interferons as anti-viral agents are, nevertheless, promising in those human cancers suspected to be of viral aetiology, or other human diseases of viral origin. In the human genome, interferon-producing genes are present. However, the amount of interferons produced is extremely small. Gamma interferons or 'immune' interferons produced by immunologically activated lymphocytes stimulate the activation of macrophages. Alpha-interferons are produced by leucocytes and more than a dozen genes have been identified using recombinant DNA technology. Beta-interferons are produced by fibroblasts. These three types of interferons inhibit proliferation of some tumour cells and can stimulate natural killer activity *in vitro*, but these effects are less pronounced *in vivo*. Perhaps the inhibition of tumours depends upon the quantity of interferons. Since interferons are species-specific, for human clinical tests, only human interferons can be employed, and these are required in large amounts. Since interferons are small proteins, it should not be too difficult to produce large quantities of human interferons in the near future by synthesizing them in the laboratory, or by inserting human interferon genes into bacteria by recombinant DNA technology, and using multiplying bacterial cells as miniature human interferon factories.

Interleukins

Stimulation of cells of the immune system by chemical mediators to fight cancer is known as 'immunotherapy'. In addition to interferons, there is another class of chemical mediators called interleukin 2 (IL-2 or T-cell growth factor) that are hormone-like substances. IL-2 can stimulate certain white blood cells into becoming cancer killers called lymphokine-activated killer (LAK) cells. The LAK cells are capable of destroying tumour cells. However, production of LAK cells requires large doses of IL-2, and this may have serious side-effects.

IL-2 can also stimulate T-lymphocytes and convert them into tumour-infiltrating lymphocytes (TIL), which attack the tumour cells and destroy them. As compared to LAK, much smaller doses of IL-2 are required for the production of TIL cells, which might minimize the side-effects. A combined therapy involves a drug called cyclophosamide, which presumably suppresses the immune system, and thus allows IL-2 to stimulate TIL more effectively to achieve tumour necrosis and elimination in mice.

The aforementioned are some of the weapons in the arsenal of therapists for the battle against cancer. Although some progress has been made towards treatment of cancer, particularly when detected early, most advanced lethal cancers are still very difficult to control or treat. Approaches to develop anti-cancer drugs are continuing. In recent years clinical interest has focussed on mechanisms of action of clinically useful nucleic acid anti-metabolites, and on methods to enhance their selective toxicity to tumours. Techniques have been developed to culture human cells in the laboratory for chemosensitivity testing and prediction of drug response, before administering the drug(s) to the cancer patients.

In addition to the aforementioned methods for treatment of cancer, new molecular genetic approaches are in the experimental stages, and should be available for diagnosis and control of cancer in the future. These methods will be briefly discussed in Chapter 19.

17

Prevention of Cancer

There is considerable evidence to suggest that about 80 per cent of human cancers are directly or indirectly influenced by environmental factors, which implies that they are, in principle, preventable. It is widely assumed that if environmental factors involved in the aetiology of human cancer can be identified, primary control, that is, prevention, is possible either through elimination or reduced exposure to such factors. Because the major human cancers vary greatly in their incidence from one country to another, they are thought to be strongly influenced by environmental factors. Epidemiological studies help identify carcinogenic agents already present in the environment, or suspected new carcinogens entering the environment, and provide necessary data for determining the degree of risk involved. A number of environmental factors have been found to be associated with human cancers (Table 17.1), and most of these factors, for example, tobacco, radiation, diet, and drugs have been discussed in previous chapters of this book. In this chapter we shall consider preventable causes of some human cancers and limitations of this approach.

Table 17.1 Environmental factors and human cancer (*Source*: R. Doll, in: *Origins of Human Cancer*, edited by H.H. Hiatt *et al.* 1977; modified).

Site	*Environmental factors*
Skin	Sunlight: ultraviolet rays; ionizing radiation; petroleum; tar products
Lung	Tobacco; air pollution; occupational inhalation of chromate, asbestos, nickel; ionizing radiation
Stomach	Diet: nitrosoamines
Colon	Diet: animal fat
Breast	Ionizing radiation; hormones; diet: animal fat?
Mouth and pharynx	Tobacco; alcohol
Oesophagus	Alcohol; tobacco, hot and strong tea (tannins?)
Liver	Alcohol; aflotoxin
Bone	Ionizing radiation: radium; strontium 90
Uterine cervix	Promiscuity; hormones
Urinary bladder	Tobacco; occupational hazards: aniline dye products
Leukaemia	Ionizing radiation; alkylating agents
Thyroid	Ionizing radiation; iodine deficiency

TOBACCO SMOKING

"Smoking is the largest single preventable cause of ill-health in the world," says the World Health Organization. There is a direct relationship between lung cancer and tobacco smoking. Tobacco smoking is also associated with cancers of the oral cavity, oesophagus, pancreas and urinary bladder, and emphysema and heart disease. Tobacco smokers are at a 10- to 50-fold higher risk of dying from lung cancer than non-smokers. Current data show that a heavy smoker who stops smoking will decrease his or her risk of cancer progressively, and after about 15 years the cancer risk will approach that of someone who has never smoked. Smoking is a contemplative and addictive habit for those who smoke, and we know such habits are very difficult to give up. Nevertheless, the quantity of tobacco smoked in the affluent countries has been falling for the past two decades. But in the Third World countries it is going up, in spite of the worldwide anti-smoking offensive. One of the main barriers to anti-smoking campaign is economic.

The tobacco industry provides livelihood to millions of people around the world, and the revenues from tax on tobacco alone contribute very large sums of money to government exchequers. For example, the revenue from tax on tobacco is almost enough to pay the salaries of all the employees as well as running costs of all the hospitals in England. Faced with such financial considerations, most governments are rather reluctant to forgo this revenue in order to support preventable medicine. From their action it would appear that they have decided on the only practical solution: to encourage the tobacco industry to design a cigarette that is relatively safe but still addictive and has a fair taxable component. Production of low-tar cigarette is a step in that direction, although, so far, the new cigarettes still pose health risks, but perhaps not as much as the old cigarettes. The purpose of the low-tar brands is to reduce the tar without affecting the taste. This mainly depends upon the filter, which captures most of the tar before it reaches the smoker's mouth. The new low-tar or ultralow-tar cigarettes may reduce the tar intake of the smoker, but the non-smoker or passive smoker in his company will inhale the same quantity of carcinogenic smoke as was the case with old cigarettes. In a way, we are trying to save the sinner, but punish the innocent!

SUNLIGHT (ULTRAVIOLET RAYS)

There is a great deal of evidence which implicates ultraviolet radiation as a prime cause of skin cancer. Skin cancer invariably develops on body areas unprotected from sunlight: the face, ears, neck, and the back of hands. Individuals, who spend long hours in bright sunlight, are at a greater risk of developing skin cancer on their exposed body areas, compared to the general population. Light-skinned (white) people are also at a greater risk of skin cancer than those with pigmented (dark) skin. Regardless of your skin colour, do not broil yourself in the sun. Prolonged sunbathing carries an increased risk for light-skinned people. Therefore, one should minimize prolonged exposure to strong sunlight, particularly at noon time.

DIET

On the basis of international variation in the incidence of cancer, and in view of altered risks of migrant populations, it has been suggested that diet is one of the major aetiologic factors in cancer of the stomach, colon, breast, and prostate.

Stomach cancer was (and still is) a major disease afflicting humans in many parts of the world. There has been considerable reduction in the incidence of stomach cancer in the United States of America and Western Europe during the last several decades. Prior to the advent of refrigeration, sizable amounts of nitrite and salt were added as food preservatives, especially to fish and meat. This is no longer necessary in the affluent countries where foods are routinely preserved under cold storage conditions. Dietary intake of nitrite and related compounds leads to the formation of nitrosoamines in the stomach. Nitrosoamines are known to cause cancer in animals, and are suspected of causing stomach and oesophagus cancers in humans. It seems that the risk of gastric cancer is lower in those people who regularly eat fresh fruits, vegetables, lettuce, and tomatoes, all sources of vitamin C, an anti-oxidant which inhibits the formation of nitrosoamines. Most people in the United States of America ingest meaningful levels of commercial anti-oxidants, which are widely used in oil, margarine, bakery products, and other substances. It has been suggested that these anti-oxidants, along with the reduction of nitrite preservatives, in the diet have contributed to the drop in the incidence of stomach cancer in the USA.

Epidemiological data suggest that a high intake of meat and animal fat, particularly beef fat, and possibly fibre deficiency are strongly associated with large bowel (colon) carcinogenesis. Dietary fat has also been implicated in the causation of human breast and prostate cancers.

As a prophylactic measure against diet-associated cancers, a 'prudent diet', which is low in animal fat from beef, egg yolk, liver (because of its extraordinarily high cholestrol content) and dairy products, but has a good supply of polyunsaturated plant fats (margarine) and oils, fresh fruit, vegetable, lettuce, tomatoes, cereals (high fibre), and légumes is recommended. The prudent diet is based on moderation; it is a varied diet, a balanced diet, which does not recommend that beef or dairy products must be eliminated or cut back drastically. But rather it recommends the use of small lean cuts of red meat (all visible fat removed) in moderation, supplemented with chicken and fish for weekly menus.

IONIZING RADIATION

There is no doubt that any form of radiation can induce cancer. Grim reminders of radiation-induced human cancers include: (1) dramatic increase in the incidence of leukaemia, and significant increase in the incidence of breast, brain, bowel, and thyroid cancers in the Japanese survivors of the atomic bomb holocaust (World War II); (2) significant increase in leukaemia in the early radiologists (who did not protect themselves when X-raying patients); and (3) tragic deaths from bone cancer of painters of luminous dials of watches (with radium-containing solution). Ionizing radiations, such as X-rays, are extensively employed for diagnostic purposes, and their maximum permissible exposures are sometimes misinterpreted to designate levels of radiation that are safe. As it turns out, all levels of radiation are unsafe in the absolute sense, no matter how small the dose may be. Therefore, preventable causes of radiation-induced cancers include necessary and minimum exposure to X-rays, mammography, or other forms of radiation for diagnostic purposes, particularly for the detection of suspected internal tumours or disease of breast, lungs, thyroid, and other tissues.

ALCOHOL, DRUGS, AND PROMISCUITY

Alcohol has been a part of the human diet for thousands of years. Even to this day, alcohol consumption remains prevalent throughout the world. There is circumstantial evidence to suggest that alcoholic beverages seem to increase the risk of cancers of the mouth, pharynx, oesophagus, and liver. Heavy drinkers who also smoke are at a particularly high risk of developing cancer of the oral cavity, not to mention the smoking-lung-cancer connection. Primary prevention of alcohol-related cancers could be achieved through campaigns directed at limiting the consumption of alcohol.

In spite of the widespread population exposure to a variety of drugs (medicinal agents) only limited knowledge regarding drug-associated human cancers has been available. This is mainly because epidemiological studies are still lacking in most cases; and the source of productive clues has been the clinical observations. Nevertheless, some drugs have been implicated in human cancer: DES (diethylstilbestrol), a synthetic estrogen, in uterine cancer; coal tar and creosote preparations in skin cancer; resperine in breast cancer; phenacetin in tumours of the kidney; chloramphenicol in leukaemia; and immunosuppressive agents in lymphomas. This is only a partial listing. Several others have been mentioned in Chapter 8. As a primary preventive measure it is recommended that inappropriate use of carcinogenic drugs should be discouraged. One should take drugs only when necessary, under the strict supervision of an experienced and 'aware' physician.

Although the relationship between viruses and human cancer is far from settled, one of the herpes viruses (Herpes Simplex Virus 2) has been implicated in cervical cancer. This virus is communicated during sexual intercourse with an infected person. Promiscuity and sexual permissiveness have greatly contributed to increased frequency of this virus and HIV (AIDS virus) both in males and females. The best advice: enjoy your married partner most and keep away from mischief!

These are then the preventable causes of some of the environmentally related cancers. As may be apparent, there are several limitations in the cancer prevention approach programme. In some cases, it may be the economic consideration, while in others, for example, in the common human cancers (stomach, colon, and breast) the precise identification of the environmental factors involved in the aetiology of cancer is still lacking. In the present circumstances, moderation is the key word. Let common sense and simple rules of safety be your best guides!

LIFESTYLE AND CANCER PREVENTION

From the standpoint of cancer prevention, the obvious questions which come to mind are: What is really safe to eat or drink? Which country is safe to live in? There is no such thing as absolute safety, whether it be diet or country; safety can be best defined in relative terms. We live in a world of Einsteinean relativity and our value judgements regarding carcinogenicity of environmental factors can at best be considered at relative standards of safety. Of course, governmental and non-governmental agencies have to determine the relative carcinogenic risks of substances already present or of new chemicals introduced into the public sector such as pesticides, food additives, food preservatives, and drugs. However, in the final analysis, the only valid prevention against cancer can best be undertaken at the individual level and each one should be responsible for oneself. Primary prevention implies avoiding exposure to recognized carcinogens or potentially carcinogenic substances in the human environment.

Individuals are at a relatively high risk of developing different cancers in different countries. For example, people in Japan, Northern and Eastern Europe are at a high risk of contracting stomach cancer. But when they emigrate to the United States of America, their descendants are not at such a high risk of developing stomach cancer, but instead they are more prone to developing cancers of colon, breast, and prostate; cancers that are prevalent in the United States' population. Therefore, each country has a certain set of environmental conditions (pollutants, diet, customs, etc.) that are relatively more conducive to the development of particular types of cancer. In all countries there is genetic variation in the population for each of the different forms of cancer. In other words, some individuals are relatively more prone to develop certain cancer(s) than others. Depending upon life-styles and exposure to certain environmental factors, only those individuals develop that cancer to which they are genetically prone. The risk factor for a cancer is determined by constant exposure to certain environmental agents. The greater the exposure to such agents, the higher the risk of developing certain cancers. Since most cancers develop after a relatively long latent period extending over a number of years, it seems that there is an additive and cumulative effect of the environmental carcinogens over a period of time. One of the simplest strategies in cancer prevention, therefore, would be to keep altering the lifestyles slightly (something not very easy to do) so that the individual is not constantly exposed to any known carcinogen or potentially carcinogenic substances in the environment so that large amounts of these substances do not accumulate in the body tissues.

13

Genetic Counselling for Hereditary Cancers

There are a number of cancer syndromes where the probands are at a markedly higher risk of developing cancer. Some of these cancer predispositions are determined by dominant or recessive (involving one or two defective genes) modes of inheritance, while in others, the cancer proneness may be polygenetically (involving several defective genes) controlled. As compared to non-cancerous hereditary diseases, different kinds of problems are encountered in the genetic counselling for hereditary cancers. Firstly, unlike many other genetic diseases, cancer is a life-threatening disease. Secondly, since most types of cancer develop at a late age, this presents a serious problem for the proband who may have to wait for many years before he or she would really know whether he or she will be affected by the disease. How does one deal with the subjects of marriage, having children, etc., during this agonizing wait-and-see period? By the time one finds out that fortunately one belongs to the unaffected progeny, then it may be too late to get married and have children. On the other hand, an individual, who may be at a high risk of cancer comes for genetic counselling after being married and having had the desired number of children, and who finds out that he has transmitted the defective gene to the progeny and thereby increased their cancer risk, might feel terribly guilty about it. These are some of the problems associated with genetic counselling of cancer probands. Nevertheless, through the process of genetic counselling, information and insight regarding the genetic nature of cancer can be provided to the persons being counselled (probands) and to their relatives who might be at a high risk of cancer, and to offer options for dealing with the occurrence and recurrence risks of the disease, with emphasis on prevention. However, the counsellor should only provide advice. The final decision to exercise the options should invariably rest with the proband. One case of autosomally dominantly inherited cancer and one of recessively inherited cancer will be discussed to illustrate the reproductive options in each case.

CANCER OF THE COLON

The predisposition towards cancer of the colon is transmitted as a dominant factor. Individuals carrying the defective gene develop polyps of the colon which, later in adult life, may develop into adenocarcinoma, a malignant tumour of the colon. The highest colon cancer risk is in individuals between 40 and 60 years of age. Those individuals who are in this category may be identified in advance by the use of colonoscopy and barium enema for the presence of polyps in the colon. If one member of the family shows colonic polyps, then all his brothers and sisters should be screened for the disease, since 50 per cent of the siblings will be affected, and the remaining 50 per cent will be unaffected. Total colectomy is the recommended treatment. When a person at a high risk of colonic cancer marries a normal person, he may be advised by a genetic counsellor about the recurrent cancer risk in the progeny. However, the persons being counselled might consider the following reproductive options: (1) they may decide to ignore the genetic risk information that 50 per cent of the children will be affected, and have any number of children; (2) they may accept the genetic risk factor, and might have one or two children, hoping they will be in the 50 per cent category of the unaffected progeny; (3) they may decide not to have any children, but elect to adopt one or more; and (4) if the affected person is a male, he may elect to be sterilized and opt for an artificial insemination for his unaffected wife, in case this option is legally and ethically open. On the other hand, if the affected person is a female, she may choose to have a sterilization job.

XERODERMA PIGMENTOSUM

Xeroderma pigmentosum is a recessive (involving two defective genes) disorder and patients suffering from this disease are at a high risk of skin cancer following exposure to strong sunlight. When two normal persons, each a carrier of a defective recessive gene for xeroderma pigmentosum, marry, the risk that they have a child affected by xeroderma pigmnentosum is one-in-four, or 25 per cent. In the recessive disorders, although the children may be at a high cancer risk, the heterozygous parent (carrying one defective gene and one normal gene at a locus) is usually not affected by the disease. By contrast, in a dominantly inherited cancer, the parent (at least one) and children (at least 50 per cent) face the cancer risk. Xeroderma pigmentosum by itself does not cause cancer, but predisposes an individual to develop skin cancer when he or she is repeatedly exposed to strong sunlight. Therefore, the xeroderma pigmentosum patients are counselled to keep away, or protect themselves, from sunlight. A relatively simple regimen of clothing and daily routines is recommended for xeroderma pigmentosum patients. They should wear large brim hats, dark glasses, long sleeved shirts, hand gloves, trousers, socks and shoes. Sports could be played by the patients afflicted by xeroderma pigmentosum at night time under artificial lights.

PROSPECTS FOR GENETIC COUNSELLING

The potential of genetic counselling has been exploited to some extent in cancers with inherited predispositions. The late stage of onset of most forms of cancer presents a serious problem in that many of the patients have already married and have had children prior to the onset of cancer. Nevertheless, certain forms of cancers may be prevented. For example, dominantly inherited cancer of the colon may be controlled through prophylactic colectomy in the patients. If such a person happens to marry late, then he may be advised by the genetic counsellor about the recurrence of colonic cancer risk in the offspring, that is, 50 per cent of the children will be at a high cancer risk. In addition to the hereditary form, the cancer of the colon also occurs sporadically or 'spontaneously' in certain individuals. Sometimes, the sporadic colonic cancer may be clustered in a family by chance and thus obfuscate the genetic issue in counselling. On the basis of pedigree analysis and the age of onset, the hereditary and sporadic forms of colon cancers may be distinguished. In the hereditary form (which is transmittable to the next generation) the age of onset of symptoms (polyps of colon) averages about 30 years, and most patients invariably die from carcinoma of the colon before the age of 50. On the other hand, in the sporadic form the symptoms may appear during middle age and the average age of death from carcinoma of the colon may be about 68 years. The sporadic form of colon cancer is not transmitted to the next generation.

In the recessively inherited cancer syndromes, one of the major problems from the standpoint of genetic counselling is the detection of heterozygous (carrier) parents, who transmit the defective genes to the progeny, of whom 25 per cent are at cancer risk. Screening and detection of carriers with the help of genetic, biochemical and molecular markers form an important area of research. If the carriers of the recessive cancer syndromes, who are usually at no personal risk of being affected, can be identified in the population, then it would be possible to advise carrier couples (before they have children) on the occurrence of cancer risk in their offspring so that they may be able to decide on their reproductive option.

Genetic counselling can become more effective when the public is educated on the inherited risks of occurrence and recurrence of cancer and how to cope with the problem. Carrier detection and early detection of cancer or the precancerous state, in some cases as early as in the foetus, would be able to provide valuable information to the genetic counsellor. When reliable detection tests are available for different forms of hereditary cancer, then through implementation of reproductive alternatives, it might be possible to considerably reduce the incidence of inherited cancers in the human population.

19

New Perspectives in Cancer Research

Cancer still remains an unresolved biological and clinical problem. The development of cancer seems to depend on an interaction between genetic and environmental factors (both intrinsic and extrinsic). Although the mechanisms of transformation of normal cells to cancer cells are not yet fully understood, it seems plausible to suggest that diverse environmental factors, such as chemical carcinogens, ionizing radiation, ultraviolet radiation, and viruses, acting singly or in concert, may affect the structure and function of certain oncogenes, or particularly regulatory genes, through mutational or epigenetic events, thereby resulting in initiation and development of cancer. Various new approaches and techniques have been developed for resolving the nature of fundamental genetics and developmental and molecular changes in the initiation and development of cancer. Some of these ideas and approaches are now discussed.

FUSION OF MALIGNANT AND NORMAL CELLS

In recent years, hybrids between malignant and normal mouse cells, or human cells, have been exploited to yield information on the nature of genetic control of malignancy. Following fusion, the hybrid cells are cultivated and then injected into appropriate animal hosts in order to test whether these hybrid cells or their descendants remain normal or give rise to tumours. In a majority of such experiments, malignancy seems to be suppressed in the hybrid cells. However, after the passage of time, the non-malignant cells, in animals, give rise to populations of cells, some of which exhibit the malignant properties. Cytological analyses have revealed that transition from the non-malignant state to the malignant state was accompanied by loss of chromosomes, particularly certain chromosomes from the normal parental complement in such hybrid cells. The implication of these findings is that normal parental cells contribute certain factors, very likely functional regulatory genes, which are impaired or lacking in the malignant cells, and these presumably suppress the malignant state in the hybrid cells between them. The suppression is removed in those descendants of the hybrid cells which have lost certain chromosomes carrying specific regulatory genes, derived from the normal parent in the hybrid cells.

The cell fusion technique has a lot of potential for future cancer research. Such research includes: (1) mapping of specific human genes whose products suppress malignancy; (2) identification of genes that code for transformation and malignant properties; (3) development of cell lines for immunological and immunotherapeutic studies through the use of hybrid cells, dubbed, 'hybridomas'; for instance, hybrid cells that inherit the ability to form antibodies (lymphocytes), and the capacity to replicate themselves indefinitely as in cancer (myeloma cells); (4) metastasis and behaviour of malignant cells; and (5) testing whether fusion between related or different kinds of malignant cells can sometimes yield hybrid cells that are non-malignant.

JUMPING GENES AND CANCER

A phenomenon relevant to the understanding of mechanisms of normal or abnormal cell differentiation may involve the so-called 'jumping genes' or 'transposable elements'. Jumping genes have the unexpected property of moving around from one region to another of a chromosome or different chromsomes, thus causing instability of gene expression and/or structural alterations at each new location. Therefore, jumping genes may play an important role in the causation of mutations and developmental changes in cells.

Jumping genes have thus far been studied intensively in the bacteria. Two types of jumping genes have been identified: (1) Insertion elements (IS) are specific DNA sequences, ranging from 800 to 1400 base pairs (equivalent to one or two genes) and (2) relatively large segments of jumping genes which confer antibiotic resistance. The IS elements can be readily inserted into bacteria, while the antibiotic-resistant jumping genes are transferred from one bacterium to another by plasmids (small pieces of extrachromosomal DNA that replicate independently in a bacterium) and viruses. The jumping genes, regardless of their size, may turn off or alter gene expression of genes or blocks of genes, adjacent to which they are inserted, and thus change certain characteristics of an organism.

There is evidence to suggest that jumping genes also exist in higher forms of life, including plants and animals. It is tempting to suggest that jumping genes may also be involved in normal and abnormal development of cells by turning off certain genes, by insertion next to these genes, or allowing them to be re-expressed after jumping genes hop to another location in the genome. Jumping genes may be directly or indirectly involved in the causation of cancer. When jumping genes transpose themselves next to the regulatory genes, that are normally involved in the prevention of cancer, and thus shut off their activity, an event (or events) which may eventually lead to the development of cancer. Alternatively, jumping genes, following attachment to viruses, may facilitate the integration of viruses in the DNA at specific sites of genetic homology, which might then permit transformation of a normal cell to a cancer cell. By employing jumping genes, plasmids and viruses, the molecular biologists are probing the nature of mutations and changes in cellular development that are relevant to the origin of cancer.

CELL DEATH AND IMMORTALITY

Living organisms do not live for ever; they die. Death is a natural part of life. Organisms die because their cells die. Therefore, cell death is closely related to the death of living organisms. So goes the dictum: what is born must die! That is the law of nature. Humans have dreamt of immortality from time immemorial. On a metaphysical and cosmic level, the body is mortal, but the soul is considered immortal. Whatever the reality, let us turn to death, in particular, cell death, and examine its consequences in an organism.

Programmed cell death (termed 'apoptosis') is an integral part of the living cells. Certain cell types must die, so that new cells can grow, proliferate and differentiate, as in a growing embryo. In the adult, the worn-out cells die so that there is a balance between cell death and cell replacement. The living cells are programmed to perform certain functions, and when their defined life-spans are over, they die at the right space and time. The genetic programme determines the survival, function as well as the mortality of normal cells. In contrast, in the cancer cells, the genetic programme appears to be impaired, so that the cell's life-span is extended, thereby partially suppressing cell death at the right time. In other words, the cell's internal death programme is disturbed. Are there specific genes involved in suppression of cell death? This is an interesting question and seems to have far-reaching implications in the human quest for immortality.

Certain oncogenes, when active, have been implicated with interference in the cell death programme. One such oncogene, known as *bcl*-2, discovered in the lymphoma tumours composed of B-cells, when activated, extends the survival of B-cells. It is known that certain immune cells die when they are deprived of cytokines (growth substances) such as interleukin-2. The prostate cells also die when they are deprived of male hormones. It would appear that an activated *bcl*-2 oncogene may block the cell death programme by stimulating cytokine-like growth substances for the rapid proliferation of B-cells. Although, an activated *bcl*-2 oncogene may interfere in the B-cell death programme, it does not make the cells cancerous. For inducing tumours, a second oncogene *myc* seems to be necessary. Presumably, cancerous growth may require the activation of two oncogenes simultaneously, but more likely in a sequential order. In addition to the oncogenic connection, are there certain other genetic events that confer on the cancer cells their ability to proliferate uncontrollably?

Single cell organisms and cancer cells have something in common: both can reproduce indefinitely, conditions permitting. One thinks of such reproduction as though immortality is the norm for both types of cells. However, this can happen only when the environmental conditions are optimal for growth. When subjected to starvation or lack of food supply, both single cell organisms and cancer cells may face the risk of extinction. Therefore, the genetic constitution and the environmental conditions determine the proliferation posture of cells. Normal human cells, however, have finite life-spans. This means that they may divide for a few dozen times, and eventually die. As mentioned earlier, normal cells have a built-in genetic programme for their life-spans. What makes the single cell organisms and cancer cells escape the programmed cell death?

It has been known for some time that single cell organisms produce an enzyme called telomerase, which adds new sequences of telomeres at the ends of DNA (chromosomes) and preserves their length. Telomeres are short strips of repeated DNA sequences (TTAGGG) found at the end of chromosomes. The telomeres have *at least* two functions: (1) they stabilize the ends of chromosomes and prevent them from degeneration and sticking together, and (2) the number of telomeres at the end of chromosomes seems to determine the number of generations a cell can divide. Every time a cell divides, a certain number of telomeres are always lost. A cell loses its ability to divide when the number of telomeres falls below a critical level. As a person ages, the number of telomeres shrink, and along with them the ability of the cells to divide. In the humans, the enzyme telomerase is not normally expressed after birth: one exception, however, is the testis. The testis apparently produce and use telomerase to rebuild telomeres for prolific production of sperm cells throughout the adult human male life. As compared to the determinate number of eggs (*ca* 400-450), which are present before birth and do not undergo any further division in a human female, the human male produces billions and billions of sperm during his lifetime. This would suggest that the telomerase gene(s) remain active in those cells which divide constantly. And single cell organisms and cancer cells belong to that category.

Recent experimental evidence provided by Calvin B. Harley and his associates indicates that human ovarian carcinoma cells express telomerase activity, as compared to normal cells, which do not. It would be interesting to find out if telomerase is produced in all types of cancer cells. If so, then it would imply that in addition to oncogenes, suppressor genes, a third class of genes, when activated, may confer on the cells a proliferation posture that appears to give them a certain degree of immortality. Of course, we know that rapid cell proliferation alone does not produce malignancy; other genetic and/or developmental changes must also occur, besides cell proliferation, for the onset of cancer.

CELL CYCLE GENES IN CANCER

There is considerable evidence to indicate that aberrations in the cell cycle machinery may contribute to uncontrollable cell division and subsequent tumour development. Cell division may be influenced by the environmental factors or by derangements of those genes involved in the regulation of cell cycle phases. The environmental factors may exert a transitory effect on the cell cycle, not necessarily affecting the cell division rate on a long-term basis, in the absence of impairment of critical genes involved in cell division. It was assumed all along that the cell cycle of a normal cell may not be substantially different from that of a cancer cell. And that all the same four phases, namely, G1, S, G2 and M or D, constitute the cell cycle machinery of normal cells as well as cancer cells (see Chapter 4). However, recent studies indicate that certain genes encoding the components of the cell cycle machinery may be potentially oncogenic. One such gene encoding a protein called cyclin D1 is apparently an oncogene. There are other genes that code for cell cycle inhibitors, and may be potential tumour suppressors. It appears that overexpression of the gene cyclin D1 may contribute to some common cancers, including those of the breast and oesophagus.

There are a number of cyclins (proteins) in the mammalian cells and D1 is one of them. The name cyclin denotes their cyclic nature, that is, their levels rise and fall in regular patterns during the cell cycle at critical intervals for regulation of cell division. At appropriate moments, enzymes called cyclin-dependent kinases (Cdks), needed to carry the cells through specific phases of the cell cycle, are activated. About half a dozen kinases have been identified, and one of them called Cdk4 is overexpressed in certain cancers. The

Cdk4 gene, which is located on chromosome 12, is a likely candidate for an oncogene. Under certain circumstances, the D1 gene and the *ras* oncogene seem to cooperate in transforming cells, thus supporting the notion that the onset of cancer requires several independent genetic changes.

Thus, it is important to investigate the cell cycle machinery, in particular, the role of cyclins and cyclin-dependent kinases (Cdks), and how they participate in regulating cell division. The components of the cell cycle would have clinical implications, as they may provide new targets for therapeutic measures. In this direction, it may be possible to inhibit the action of D1 or other cyclins to block the uncontrolled cell division and growth. Since components of the cell cycle deteriorate as a tumour progresses towards the malignant state, it might be possible to use this knowledge on the cell cycle to monitor the patient's cancer status.

REGULATORY GENES AND SUPPRESSOR GENES

Cancer is a genetic disease probably involving the impairment of regulatory controls that apparently trigger off tumour initiation and development. The basic genetic information for the induction of tumours seems to be present in the normal cells of higher organisms. This tumour-inducing genetic information, called *Tu* or *onc* genes, is normally controlled in an organism by the regulatory genes (*R*-genes) that suppress the expression of oncogenes. Sometimes the tumour suppressor genes have been called anti-oncogenes. One such tumour suppressor gene, called p53 (p stands for protein with a molecular weight of 53 kilodaltons) and discovered back in 1979, was found in association with tumour-causing viruses.The tumour suppressor gene has been mapped on human chromosome 17 position p13, written as 17p13. Subsequently, mutated forms of p53 have been found in both inherited and spontaneous human cancers. As it turns out, p53 is the most commonly mutated suppressor gene in as many as 50 per cent of the human cancers. These include cancers of the colon, lung, breast, stomach, skin, ovary, liver, oesophagus, brain, bladder, cervix, larynx, pancreas, prostate, and thyroid. The suppressor gene p53 is involved in the regulation of growth in the normal cells; only its mutated forms are associated with cancer and may be involved in promoting abnormal cell growth. How does p53 suppress tumour development?

Although precise mechanisms of p53 action have not yet been entirely understood, it appears that p53 controls cell division and growth, and can stimulate programmed cell death in response to DNA damage. In other words, p53 keeps a tight control on cell division and growth, and thereby suppresses uncontrolled growth that might lead to cancer development. The tumour suppressor gene p53 thus may control the activity and expression of oncogenes that might otherwise lead to tumour formation.

In addition to p53, a number of other tumour suppressor genes have been identified. These include tumour suppressor genes for retinoblastoma (*Rb*) located on human chromosome 13p14, adenomatous polyposis (*APC*) mapped on chromosome 5q21, breast cancer (*BRCA1*) located on 17q21, neuroblastoma (*NB1*) on chromosome 1p36, and a gene that codes for a p16 protein. Among these, p16 is currently under active study. This tumour suppressor gene is located on human chromosome 9p21. Mutant forms of p16 have been detected in a variety of human cancers, including those of the breast, bladder, kidney, and melanomas. The protein from p16 gene binds itself to an enzyme known as cyclin-dependent kinase 4 (Cdk4), one of the several Cdks involved in cell division. One of the Cdk4 cyclin partner genes, cyclin D1, can act as an oncogene, when uncontrolled. These findings suggest that suppressor genes and oncogenes act in concert to maintain balanced growth and development under normal circumstances. Mutant forms of suppressor genes can have disastrous consequences for growth and carry a risk of cancer development.

The study on tumour suppressor genes will open up new therapeutic options. One includes restoring a normal copy of suppressor genes (for example, p53 or p16) in the human tumours by gene transfer. Another approach would be to correct the mutational mistakes by substitution of changed amino acids and correcting the configuration of the p53 or p16 proteins, so that they perform their normal regulatory functions. However, it may be premature to assume that restoring one gene to its normal form (function) in a tumour would lead to tumour regression and normal growth. It may turn out that the gene therapy may involve restoring two or more critical normal genes in a tumour, which are essential for normal growth and development. The best approach would be to restore critical suppressor genes at an early stage of tumour development, long before the onset of the malignant state.

GENOME STRUCTURE AND MAPPING

Knowledge about the structure and function of the human genome is a prerequisite for gene therapy in cancer. The human genome, that is, the genetic information in the human germ cells (the egg and the sperm cells) contains 3×10^9 base pairs (bp) of DNA. This means that there are some 3 billion base pairs in a human genome, which correspond to 750 megabytes of information in computer language. Two approaches have been employed to decipher this genetic information. One involves the analysis of the sequences of bases in the structure of genes that code for specific proteins for specific functions. The other deals with the location and order of genes on the 23 human chromosomes. Sequencing of DNA would also permit an understanding of control of regulation through structural analysis of regulatory or suppressor genes. Thus, DNA sequencing would enable us to gain an insight into how genetic information involved in the control and expression of the structure and the function of cells is encoded in the DNA molecule. The discovery of DNA-cleaving enzymes (restriction enzymes) in 1970 made it possible to sequence DNA segments of varying lengths. Site-specific restriction enzymes will cut DNA at specific sites (by recognition of the bases in the DNA string) and yield smaller or larger segments of DNA. The sequence of the DNA fragments, whose terminal ends have been marked, can be accomplished by chemical means.

One of the efficient methods, known as the chain termination sequencing technique, has been routinely employed for determining the sequence of DNA bases. This method is based on enzymatic DNA synthesis carried out in a test tube (*in vitro*). A single DNA strand is provided as a template for building a second strand in a test tube containing the necessary ingredients and enzymes necessary for DNA synthesis. By employing artificial chain-terminating variants of the normal DNA precursor molecule, individual sequences ranging from 1000 to 10,000 base pairs could be determined. Although this method was useful for determining the base sequences of smaller DNA fragments, newer techniques had to be developed for the analysis of the large human genome consisting of some 3 billion base pairs.

By employing restriction enzymes, DNA can be chopped up into fragments of different sizes. Differences between these pieces are called restriction fragment length polymorphisms or just RFLPs (pronounced rif-lips). For a given genome, there is a characteristic catalogue of RFLPs, each with a specific sequence of bases. RFLPs provide a valuable collection of genetic markers along the length of a chromosome, and thus allow us to track the location of a normal or defective gene. By employing RFLPs, along with PCR (polymerase chain reaction)-based molecular markers called RAPDs (random amplified polymorphic DNAs), researchers have been able to map a large number of genes on human chromosomes. Once the location of a normal or defective gene has been determined, it is then possible to isolate and clone that specific gene for structural analysis of bases. After a gene has been cloned, it is then possible to introduce it in a viral or bacterial vector for genetic engineering and gene transfer.

GENETIC ENGINEERING AND CANCER

Development of certain techniques in molecular biology, during the past decades, has made it possible to break and rejoin segments of DNA in a variety of different ways. With the advent of recombinant DNA technology, it is now possible to introduce genetic material from one individual to another within a species, or in totally unrelated species. DNA is isolated from chromosomes, and cleaved into fragments that may contain one or several genes. The cleaving enzymes break DNA into pieces that have sticky ends, so that it can be joined in a variety of different ways. The cleaved genes are then introduced into a circular chromosome of bacterial plasmid. The multiplying bacteria rapidly produce thousands of copies of the gene spliced into the plasmids. The plasmids carrying this new piece of genetic information are then used as vectors, to transfer this genetic information (genes) into the host cell DNA. In humans gene cloning and transfer have been accomplished with the help of certain viruses, in particular modified (harmless) retroviruses.

Genetic engineering, or manipulation of genes, is a revolutionary new experimental approach for attempting modification of the genetic content of a cell, whether normal or cancerous. Therefore, genetic engineering technology will have the greatest bearing on the future of cancer research. The ability to manipulate genes, or parts of genes, within a cell, or the introduction of desirable genes from one individual to another or one organism to another, and to change the character, behaviour and attributes of living cells has far-reaching possibilities for the future of mankind. Among other things, genetic engineering offers prospects for modifying or controlling harmful genes in plants, animals and humans. Since cancer is a genetic disease, genetic engineering may hopefully provide means to either remove those genes involved in malignancy or introduce normal genes that are involved in the suppression of cancer. However, there are limitations to gene therapy. The techniques for gene therapy are expensive, and may have to be repeated several times before the gene integrates at the *right place* in the DNA. Another problem is that it is not certain how many copies of a gene are inserted and where they end up in the genome; perhaps on one or several chromosomes. In that event, certain host genes may be activated or shut off by the position effect of the introduced gene(s), and thus may cause growth abnormalities, including cancer. It is also possible that some genes, when transferred from one individual to another, may integrate at specific sites because of their affinity to other genes in the genome, thus modifying specific traits of normal or cancer cells. It is a paradox that, on the one hand, gene therapy offers prospects of curing or controlling cancer, and, on the other, it evokes certain possible dangers by shutting off suppressor genes or turning on oncogenes. In this respect, gene therapy may represent a double-edged sword that can cut through cancer as well as normal cells, destroying one at the expense of the other. Therefore, manipulation of genes should be carried out cautiously and carefully, and according to the current guidelines and regulations prescribed by governments, and those experiments considered inappropriate, because of their potential biohazards to mankind, should not be initiated. Genes are the building blocks of life, they should be first fully investigated and understood on the molecular level, and then handled with respect before transferring them to an old territory or a new one in search of a homeland.

20

Origin and Evolution of Cancer Genes

THE REPLICATOR

In this chapter I shall present speculations on the origin of cancer genes, and argue that these genes are part of the evolutionary history of the multicellular organisms. It is probable that life originated on Planet Earth some 3 billion years ago (some estimates put that figure close to 4 billion). The origin of the self-perpetuating replicator molecule DNA (although the first transitional replicator could have been an RNA entity or even an autocatalytic protein polymer) was critical to the development and evolution of life on earth. Even though the genetic dictionary contains only four letters of the alphabet A (adenine), T (thymine), G (guanine), and C (cytsine), there is enormous potential, depending upon the arrangements of letters, for genetic diversity and the origin of species. The first putative pre-life organisms may have been relatively simple RNA or DNA viruses that could exist in the early hostile environment. However, most of the pre-life organisms were probably wiped out as the environment changed rapidly. But some genetic variants of virus-like particles may have taken to the parasitic mode of existence when the first single cell life organisms originated. Although it is equally likely that viruses, having a dual existence (alive when inside a living cell, and inert when outside a living cell), could have evolved subsequently by the excision of cellular genes.

Two of the prime life functions for genetic continuity were reproduction and perpetuation of the organisms. Since development of dimorphic sex took place much later in the evolutionary scale, initially reproduction occurred by cloning, that is, a one-cell primitive organism reproduced by spontaneous division called binary fission into two (common among bacteria and protozoa), along with the replication of the hereditary molecule DNA. In these simple organisms the genetic programme apparently did not contain genes that would regulate cell division stringently. These organisms reproduced rapidly, almost without restraint, so long as the environmental conditions (including food supply) were conducive. When the conditions were adverse, the organisms failed to reproduce and died. Because of the inherent nature of the replicator molecule, new variants are produced by mutations to meet new challenges in a changing environment. Besides, relatively simple sexual reproduction by conjugation in the one-cell organisms probably originated to generate additional genetic variability by recombinational events for the survival of the organisms. As life evolved from a unicellular to multicellular form, three-dimensional growth and differentiation were subsequently established as essential processes, in addition to cell reproduction, for the further development and evolution of specialized forms of higher organisms. I postulate that it was during the transition from unicellular to multicellular organisms that the incipient cancer genes evolved and continue to evolve from cell reproduction genes. However, for normal growth these genes had to be regulated. Thus, cell reproduction, three-dimensional growth and differentiation must proceed in a balanced and coordinated fashion for the normal development and functioning of a complex multicellular organism. Along with the differentiated states, also evolved genes in the replicator molecule whose products were necessary for the formation of specialized tissues and organs in the higher organisms.

ONTOGENY OF CANCER GENES

In the ever-changing environment, nothing remains constant. Ever since the origin of life some 3 billion years ago, the DNA molecule has undergone changes not only in size in different organisms, but also in its organization (sequences of bases) of the universal bases A, T, G, and C. Different segments of DNA perfomed different functions. Certain segments of DNA coded for specific structural proteins, others for specific enzymes, and still others regulated the expression of structural genes. Besides, there are large segments of the total DNA in the genome which are repetitive (sometimes called junk DNA) and may not have a detectable or measurable function. Perhaps some of the regulatory genes may reside in this region. Clearly, some genes control the expression of other genes. However, gene expression is also strongly influenced by the environment, both intrinsic and extrinsic. Changes in the structural organization of genes that are heritable (mutations) have played a very important role in the origin of species. In a changing environment, certain mutants have a selective advantage as the new variants are better adapted to the new environment, as compared to their progenitors. However, all through evolution, genes promoting rapid cell division were retained in the cellular organisms. These genes are important for their survival and development. These genes are turned on during stage-specifc bursts of cell division, for example, during embryonic development and cellular repair, and then turned off or remain suppressed during most of the normal development of an organism. These genes or similar ones may also be responsible for the attainment of an organ-specific cell number during growth and development.

The human body, on an average, consists of some 100 trillion (10^{14}) cells. There are about 100 cell types in different organs/tissues in a human body. It is assumed that the same number (100) of cellular proto-oncogenes may be present in the human genome, and in each cell type these genes (crucial for cell division and growth) are controlled/regulated by cell/tissue-specific regulatory or suppressor genes, which may be different for different cell types, although some occasional sharing may not be uncommon. This means that each tissue/organ has its own intrinsic cell division rate and limit. Impairment or loss of suppressor genes in tissues would lead to unrestrained cell division, which may initiate the pre-cancerous state. A number of additional genetic and/or epigenetic changes would be necessary for the development of cancer.

The implication of this discussion is that cells of multicellular organisms contain genetic information for the initiation and development of cancer. Although it is difficult to determine when the constellation of genes involved in cancer formation originated, I postulate that this was probably a biphasic development in time and space accompanying the transition from unicellular to multicellular organisms. It is conjectured that the origin of stable cell reproduction genes may have taken place some 3-2 billion years ago in the unicellular organisms, but the genes involved in development and differentiation may have originated much later, perhaps 2-1 billion years ago, along with the three-dimensional development of multicellular organisms. According to this concept, the cellular genes involved in cancer (oncogenes) are ancient and have been part of the evolutionary history of higher organisms. During the evolutionary process, a rigid infrastructure of controlling elements, the regulatory or suppressor genes, has been built around those oncogenes, which, when uncontrolled, might lead to initiation and development of cancer. The initiation process may be relatively short, and may involve one or two genetic changes. However, the development process may involve a number of additional genetic and/or epigenetic changes over a period of time, sometimes extending to many years. The impairment of suppressor genes may, in part, depend on the lifestyle of an individual.

Where do retroviruses and oncogenes fit in this picture? That is an interesting question and has received a lot of attention. As mentioned in the beginning of this chapter, virus-like particles may have been the first non-living/living organisms that inhabited Planet Earth. But their later development was subjected to the existence of living cells. The transfer of genes between viruses and cells may have contributed to the origin of environmentally conditioned genetic engineering in those early days of our planet. Therefore, genetic engineering has probably existed in nature for a long time as a process promoting the origin of new genotypes and forms of life. Among others, the oncogenes are those notorious genes that are somehow involved in the carcinogenesis process, and can be transferred from cells to viruses and vice versa. Once active, the oncogenes turn into aggressive genes that take over the cellular machinery and convert normal cells into cancer cells, which become invasive, and eventually destroy the normal neighbouring cells. But the genes that have turned into oncogenes are, under normal circumstances, not deleterious, and may still perform some stage-specific useful functions. That is why these proto-oncogenes or cellular oncogenes have been retained in the genetic programme of the multicellular organsims over billions of years and are part of their evolutionary history.

It is indeed ironic that as long as there are normal cells that are capable of cell division, there remains a possibility that they might become cancerous in the multicellular organisms. Therefore, it is essential to identify potentially cancer-inducing genes, their products, and regulatory or suppressor genes that control their expression, and genes that enhance tumour development and induce aggressive cellular behaviour. In this direction, an understanding of the processes involved in cell reproduction, differentiation, and behaviour is critical for cancer research.

Epilogue

We have come a long way in terms of understanding the structure and function of normal cells. However, many aspects of the growth and differentiation of cells, whether normal or cancerous, have not yet been well comprehended. What transforms a normal cell into a cancer cell still remains an enigma. Does it involve changes in the structure of suppressor genes as well as oncogenes? How many genetic and epigenetic changes are required for the development of a specific cancer, say, lung cancer? We are unable to answer these questions with any degree of certainty. Perhaps to shift the emphasis, we might ask: What protects a normal cell from becoming cancerous? I think this last question would be more relevant to our understanding of normal cellular mechanisms that regulate cell reproduction and differentiation in an orderly way. In this direction the cancer cells, which are essentially aberrant normal cells may provide some answers to the regulation and maintenance of normal growth and development. Thus, the functionless cancer cells may, after all, serve as useful mutant cells for understanding principles of normal growth. This concept also entails implications for the prevention of cancer.

What prevents a normal cell from being transformed into a cancer cell? The search for genes that suppress tumour formation has been going on for a long time. In recent years, several tumour suppressor genes have been identified. These genes apparently regulate the expression of cellular proto-oncogenes that are inherent in the human genome. Under normal circumstances, the proto-oncogenes perform certain normal functions, and may be involved in cell division and growth at specific periods of development and cellular repair. However, the impairment of tumour suppressor genes by mutational events may release the proto-oncogenes from suppression and may trigger off the initiation phase of carcinogenesis. However, initiation alone does not lead to tumour development. Additional genetic and/or developmental changes are required for cancerous growth. All these changes in the tumour suppressor genes as well as other genes involved in the tumour development normally do not occur in quick succession, but rather take place over a period of time, sometimes extending from 5 to 15 years in humans. In other words, there is normally a long latent period from the initiation phase to the development of malignancy. Besides, all the normal cells that are transformed may not necessarily reach the final cancerous state. In fact, most of the early transformants are probably knocked out by the body's immune system. It is only those rare transformants that somehow escape the stringent defence mechanism which may proceed further when additional genetic/epigenetic changes occur in them. This may eventually lead to tumour development. Therefore, there are several points of reference in the chain of events from a normal cell to a cancer cell that offer opportunities for prevention and treatment of cancer.

According to this line of thinking, we should focus on those environmental factors, in particular, potentially carcinogenic substances, that impair or mutate the tumour suppressor genes. In my opinion, recognition of those environmental factors involved in the initiation of cancer, in particular, the three major human cancers of lung, breast and large intestine responsible for about half the cancer deaths, may help lower the cancer incidence and bring tremendous relief to human suffering. Therefore, we should aim at minimizing the levels of known carcinogens and other potentially carcinogenic chemicals in our environment, and thereby reduce human cancer risks.

Where do we go from here? As our twentieth century comes to a close and we enter the twenty-first century, it would be useful to characterize the tumour suppressor genes, oncogenes, and other tumour enhancer genes, on the one hand, and to recognize and reduce those environmental factors that seem to impair them, on the other. This may not eliminate human cancer altogether, but at least, it may be possible to reduce the cancer incidence in the human populations. Some hereditary cancers, such as xeroderma pigmentosum, causing skin cancer, are preventable by avoiding exposure to sunlight. However, other hereditary cancers, including those of colon and eye (retinoblastoma), may require precise understanding of specific intrinsic and extrinsic environmental factors triggering off these cancers. Alternatively, gene therapy may be required to replace the defective tumour suppressor genes with normal counterparts in such cancers.

Along with these prevention strategies, screening and detection of cancer would hopefully offer reasonably good approaches for treatment and cure of cancer. In the final analysis, cancer prevention can be carried out, at best, at the individual level. Let common sense and the golden rule of moderation be the best guides for your lifestyle, wherever you live on this Planet Earth. After all, when we look back towards the ancient past, life probably originated in a hostile environment; it has survived the vagaries of nature and other catastrophes during the last 3-4 billion years, and has evolved in a diversity of magnificent forms, including the highest evolved species, the *Homo sapiens*. Cancer is an ancient disease, and has probably existed for a long time even in the earlier forms of life, much before the apes or the humans came into existence. However, the incidence of this disease may have been low in the early humans. Things probably changed rapidly following urbanization. Epidemiological data show that there has been an increase in human cancer incidence following industrialization. By irresponsible use of pesticides, herbicides, food additives (preservatives or colouring agents), and spewing poisonous and hazardous pollutants into the environment, we are not only increasing the risks of human cancer and other diseases, but also compromising the very existence of life on our precious planet.

Select Bibliography

Aaronson, S.A., Bishop, J.M., Sugimura, T., Terada, M., Toyoshima, K. and Vogt, P.K.,1987, *Oncogenes and Cancer*, Japan Scientific Societies Press, Tokyo.

Adams, D., Dimitrijevic, N. and Schartl, M., 1993, Tumor suppression in *Xiphophorus* by an accidentally acquired promoter, *Science*, **259**:816-819.

Ahuja, M.R., 1965, Genetic control of tumor formation in higher plants, *Quart. Rev. Biol.*, **40**:329-340.

Ahuja, M.R., 1968, An hypothesis and evidence concerning the genetic components controlling tumor formation in *Nicotiana*, *Mol. Gen. Genet.*, **103**:176-184.

Ahuja, M.R., 1979, On the nature of genetic change as an underlying cause for the origin of neoplasms. In: *Antiviral Mechanisms in the Control of Neoplasia*, Chandra, P. (ed.), Plenum Press, New York, pp. 17-37.

Ahuja, M.R., 1996, Genetic nature of a non-tumor mutant isolated from a tumour-prone amphidiploid, *Nicotiana-glauca-langsdorffii* (GGLL): A critical assessment, *Heredity*, **76**: 335-345.

Ahuja, M.R. and Anders, A., 1976, A genetic concept of the origin of cancer, based in part upon studies of neoplasms in fishes, *Prog. Exp. Tumour Res.*, **20**:380-397.

Ahuja, M.R. and Anders, A., 1977, Cancer as a problem of gene regulation. In: *Recent Advances in Cancer Research: Cell Biology, Molecular Biology, and Tumor Virology*, vol. 1, Gallo, R.C. (ed.), CRC Press, Cleveland, Ohio, pp. 103-117.

Ahuja, M.R. and Dempster, E.R., 1983, Some statistical considerations on the mutational/epigenetic origin of human cancer, XV International Congress of Genetics, Part I, Oxford University Press, New Delhi, p. 53.

Anders, A. and Anders, F., 1978, Etiology of cancer as studied in platyfish-swordtail system, *Biochem. Biophys. Acta,* **516**:61-95.

Anders, F., 1991, Contributions of the Gordon-Kosswig melanoma system to the present concept of neoplasia, *Pigment Cell Res.*, **3**:7-29.

Anonymous, 1986, *Cancer Biology -- Readings from Scientific American*, Introduction by Errol C. Friedberg, W.H. Freeman and Company, New York.

Anonymous, 1993, *Cancer: Facts and Figures – 1993.* American Cancer Society, Atlanta, Georgia.

Anonymous, 1992, *Cancer Risk Report – Prevention and Control*, 1992, American Cancer Society, Atlanta, Georgia.

Armstrong, B. and Doll, R., 1975, Environmental factors and cancer incidence and mortality in different countries, with special reference to dietary practices, *Int. J. Cancer,* **15**:617-631.

Barr, P. J. and Tomei, L.D., 1994, Apoptosis and its role in human disease, *Bio/Technology*, **12**:487-493.

Baserga, R. (ed.), 1971, *The Cell Cycle and Cancer*, Marcel Decker, New York.

Bauer, K.H., 1928, *Mutationtheorie der Geschwulst-Entstehung. Übergang von Körper-zellen in Geschwulstzellen durch Gen-Änderung (Mutation Theory for the Origin of Tumors — Transition from Somatic Cells to Tumor Cells through Genetic Change)*, Verlag von Julius Springer, Berlin.

Berenbaum, I., 1974, *Carcinogenesis as a Biological Process*, North-Holland Publishing Company, Amsterdam.

Bertelsen, A.H. *et al.*, 1995, Tumor suppressor genes: Prospects for cancer therapy, *Bio/Technology*, **13**:127-131.

Bishop, J.M., Rowley, J.D. and Greaves, M. (eds.), 1984, *Genes and Cancer*, Alan R. Liss, New York.

Boice, J.D. and Fraumeni, J.J. (eds). 1984, *Radiation Carcinogenesis: Epidemiology and Biological Significance,* Raven Press, New York.

Boring, C.C., Squires, T. and Tong, T., 1993. *Cancer Statistics*, American Cancer Society, Atlanta, Georgia.

Boveri, Theodore, 1914, *Zur Frage der Entstehung maligner Tumoren* (*The Origin of Malignant Tumors*). Verlag von Gustav Fischer, Jena.

Braun, A.C., 1969, *The Cancer Problem*, Columbia University Press, New York.

Braun, A.C., 1974, *The Biology of Cancer*, Addison-Wesley, Reading, Massachusetts.

Braun, A.C., 1981, An epigenetic model for the origin of cancer, *Quart. Rev. Biol.*, **56**:33-60.

Busch, H., 1974, *The Molecular Biology of Cancer*, Academic Press, New York.

Cairns, J., 1978, *Cancer: Science and Society*. W.H. Freeman and Company, San Francisco.

Carney, D. and Sikora, K. (eds.), 1990, *Genes and Cancer,* John Wiley and Sons, New York.

Chandra, P. (ed.), 1979, *Antiviral Mechanisms in the Control of Neoplasia*, Plenum Press, New York.

Chumakor, I.M. *et al.*, 1995, A YAC contig map of human genome, *Genome Directory, Nature Suppl*, **377**: 175-297.

Comings, D.E., 1973, A general theory of carcinogenesis, *Proc. Nat. Acad. Sci. USA*, **70**:3324-3328.

Counter, C.M., Hirte, H.W., Bacchetti, S. and Harley, C.B., 1994, Telomerase activity in human ovarian carcinoma, *Proc. Nat. Acad. Sci. USA*, **91**:2900-2904.

Croce, C.M. and Koprowski, H., 1978, The genetics of human cancer, *Sci. American*, **238**:117-125.

Cullota, E. and Koshland, D.E., 1993, P53 sweeps through cancer research, *Science*, **262**:1958-1961.

Curtis, H.J., 1971, Genetic factors in aging, *Adv. Genetics*, **16**:305-324.

De Roberts, E.D. and De Roberts, E.M.F., 1987, *Cell and Molecular Biology*, Lea and Febiger, Philadelphia.

De Vita, V.T., Hellman, S. and Rosenberg, S.A. (eds.), 1989, *Cancer – Principles and Practices of Oncology*, 3rd edition, J.B. Lippincott Company, Philadelphia.

Doll, R., 1967, *Prevention of Cancer: Pointers from Epidemiology*, The Nuffield Provincial Hospitals' Trust, London.

Doll, R. and Peto, R., 1981, *The Causes of Cancer*, Oxford University Press, New York.

Duesberg, P.H., 1985, Activated proto-oncogenes: sufficient or necessary for cancer? *Science*, **228**:669-677.

Ephrussi, B., 1972, *Hybridization of Somatic Cells*, Princeton University Press, Princeton.

Essex, M., Todaro, G. and zur Hausen, H. (eds.), 1980, *Viruses in Naturally Occurring Cancers*, Cold Spring Harbor, New York.

Fialkow, P.J., 1976, Clonal origin of human tumors, *Cancer Reviews*, **458**:283-321.

Foulds, L., 1975, *Neoplastic Development*, Academic Press, New York.

Fraumeni, J.F. (ed.), 1975, *Persons at High Risk of Cancer: An Approach to Cancer Etiology and Control*, Academic Press, New York.

Friedberg, E.C. 1985, *DNA Repair*, W.H. Freeman and Company, New York.

Friend, S.H., 1993, Genetic models for studying cancer susceptibility, *Science,* **259**:774-775.

Gallo, R.C. (ed.), 1977, *Recent Advances in Cancer Research: Cell Biology, Molecular Biology, and Tumor Virology,* vols. 1 and 2, CRC Press, Cleveland, Ohio.

Gordon, M., 1958, A genetic concept for the origin of melanoma. In: Genetic Concept for the Origin of Cancer, *Ann. N.Y. Acad. Sci.*, **71**:1213-1222.

Harris, C.C. and Autrup, H.N. (eds.), 1983, *Human Carcinogenesis,* Academic Press, New York.

Hayflick, L., 1965, The limited *in vitro* lifetime of human diploid strains, *Exp. Cell Res.,* **25**:585-621.

Heidelberger, C., 1975, Chemical carcinogenesis, *Ann. Rev. Biochemistry,* **44**:49-121.

Heston, H.E., 1976, Genetic aspects of human cancer, *Adv. Cancer Res.*, **23**:1-21.

Hiatt, H.H., Watson, J.D. and Winsten, J.A. (eds.), 1977, *Origins of Human Cancer*, Cold Spring Harbor, New York.

Hilgers, J. and Sluyser, M. (eds.), 1981, *Mammary Tumors in the Mouse*, Elsevier North-Holland, Amsterdam.

Hinds, P.W., Dowdy, S.F., Eaton, E.N., Arnold, A. and Weinberg, R.A., 1994, Function of a human cyclin gene as an oncogene, *Proc. Nat. Acad. Sci. USA*, **91**:709-713.

Holland, J., Frei, E., Bast, R., Kuff, D., Morton, D. and Weichelbaum, R. (eds.), 1993, *Cancer Medicine*, 3rd edition, Lea and Febiger, Philadelphia.

Hollstein, M., Sidransky, D., Vogelstein, B. and Harris, C.C., 1991, P53 mutations in human cancer, *Science,* **253**:49-52.

Hueper, W.C., 1966, *Occupational and Environmental Cancers of the Respiratory System*, Springer Verlag, Berlin and New York.

Hueper, W.C., 1969, *Occupational and Environmental Cancers of the Urinary System*, Yale University Press, New Haven.

Kahn, P. and Graf, T. (eds.), 1987, *Oncogenes and Growth Control*, Springer Verlag, Berlin and New York.

Kanungo, M.S., 1980, *Biochemistry of Aging*, Academic Press, London.

Kato, H. and Schull, W.J., 1982, Studies of the mortality of A-bomb survivors: Mortality, 1950-1978, Part I, Cancer Mortality, *Radiation Res.*, **90**:395-432.

Kauffman, S.A., 1993, *The Origins of Order*, Oxford University Press, New York.

Kellermann, G., Shaw, C.R. and Luyten-Kellermann, M., 1973, Aryl hydrocarbon hydroxylase inducibility and bronchial carcinoma, *New England J. Med.*, **289**: 971-973.

Klein, G. (ed.), 1990, *Tumor Suppressor Genes*, Marcel Decker, New York.

Knudson, A.G., 1977, Genetics and etiology of human cancer, *Adv. Human Genetics*, **8**:1-66.

Knudson, A.G., 1993, Antioncogenes and human cancer, *Proc. Nat. Acad. Sci. USA.*, **90**:10914-10921.

Lewin, B., 1990, *Genes IV*, Oxford University Press, New York.

Lloyd, C.W. and Rees, D.A. (eds.), 1981, *Cellular Control in Differentiation*, Academic Press, New York.

Lloyd, D., Poole, R.K. and Edwards, S.W., 1982, *The Cell Division Cycle*, Academic Press, New York.

Lynch, H.T., Lynch, P.M. and Lynch, J.F., 1979, Genetic counselling and cancer. In: *Genetic Counselling – Psychological Dimensions,* Kessler, S. (ed)., Academic Press, New York, pp. 221-241.

McCann, J. and Ames, B.N., 1976, Detection of carcinogens as mutagens in Salmonella-microsome test: assay of 300 chemicals – discussion, *Proc. Nat. Acad. Sci. USA*, **73**:950-954.

Merson, M.H., 1993, Slowing the spread of HIV: agenda for the 1990s, *Science*, **260**:1266-1268.

Miller, D., 1992, Human gene therapy comes of age, *Nature*, **237**:455-460.

Mintz, Beatrice and Fleischman, R.A., 1981, Teratocarcinoma and other neoplasms as developmental defects in gene expression, *Adv. Cancer Res.*, **34**:211-278.

Mitelman, F., 1986, Clustering of breakpoints to specific chromosomal regions in human neoplasia: A survey of 5345 cases, *Hereditas*, **104**:113-119.

Mulligan, R.C., 1993, The basic science of gene therapy, *Science*, **260**:926-932.

Mulvihill, J.J., Miller, R.W. and Fraumeni, J.F. (eds.), 1977, *Genetics of Human Cancer*, Raven Press, New York.

Nevers, P. and Saedler, H., 1977, Transposable genetic elements as agents of gene instability and chromosomal rearrangements, *Nature*, **268**:109-115.

Olson, M.V., 1993, The human genome project, *Proc. Nat. Acad. Sci. USA*, **90**:4338-4344.

Orgel, L.E., 1973., Aging of clones of mammalian cells, *Nature*, **243**:441-445.

Orgel, L.E., 1992, Molecular replication, *Nature*, **358**:203-209.

Pierce, G.B., Shikes, R. and Fink, L.M., 1978, *Cancer: A Problem of Developmental Biology*, Prentice-Hall, Engelwood Cliffs, New Jersey.

Pimentel, E., 1989, *Oncogenes*, CRC Press, Boca Raton, Florida.

Plautz, G.E. *et al.*, 1993, Immunotherapy of malignancy by *in vivo* gene transfer into tumors, *Proc. Nat. Acad. Sci. USA*, **90**:4645-4649.

Prescott, D.M., 1973, *Cancer: The Misguided Cell,* The Bobbs-Merril Co., New York.

Ptashne, M., 1986, Gene regulation by proteins acting nearby and at a distance, *Nature*, **322**:697-701.

Rabbitts, T.H., 1994, Chromosomal translocations in human cancer, *Nature,* **372**:143-149.

Richards, V., 1978, *The Wayward Cell Cancer*, University of California Press, Berkeley.

Rowley, J.D., 1984, The biological implications of consistent chromosome rearrangements, *Cancer Res.*, **44**:3159-3168.

Sachs, L.,1986, Growth, differentiation and reversal of malignancy, *Sci. American,* **254**:40-47.

Schultz, J., 1958, Malignancy and genetics of somatic cell. In: Genetic Concept for the Origin of Cancer, *Ann. N.Y. Acad. Sci.*, **71**:994-1008.

Searle, C.E., 1976, Chemical Carcinogenesis, American Chemical Society, Washington.

Setlow, R.B., 1978, Repair deficient human disorders and cancer, *Nature*, **271**:713-717.

Shapiro, J.A., 1983, *Mobile Genetic Elements,* Academic Press, New York.

Sluyser, M. (ed.), 1990, *Molecular Biology of Cancer Genes,* Ellis Horwood, New York.

Stanbridge, E.J., 1976, Suppression of malignancy in human cells, *Nature,* **260**:17-20.

Tomatis, L. (ed.), 1990, *Cancer: Causes, Occurrence and Control*, International Agency for Research on Cancer, Lyon.

Varmus, H., 1987, Reverse transcriptase, *Sci. American*, **257**:56-64.

Varmus, H., 1988, Retroviruses, *Science,* **240:**1427-1435.

Vaziri, H., Dragowska, W., Allsopp, R.C., Thomas, T.E., Harley, C.B., and Lansdorp, P.M., 1994, Evidence for a mitotic clock in human hemoatopoietic cells: loss of telomeric DNA with age, *Proc. Nat. Acad. Sci. USA,* **91**:9857-9860.

Wakabayashi, T. *et al.,* 1983, Studies on the mortality of A-Bomb survivors, Part III, Incidence of cancer in 1958-78, based on the tumor registry, Nagasaki. *Radiation Res.,* **93**:112-146.

Weinberg, R.A. (ed.), 1989, *Oncogenes and the Molecular Origins of Cancer,* Cold Spring Harbor, New York.

Weiss, R., Teich, N., Varmus, H. and Coffin, C. (eds.), 1982, *RNA Tumor Viruses*, Cold Spring Harbor, New York.

Weiss, R.A., 1993, How does HIV cause AIDS?, *Science*, **260**:1273-1278.

White, R. and Caskey, T., 1988, The human as an experimental system in molecular genetics, *Science*, **240**:1483-1488.

Whitney, J.B. and Lemoreux, M.L., 1982, Transposable elements controlling genetic instability in mammals, *J. Heredity*, **73:** 12-18.

Williams, C.J. (ed.)., 1990, *Cancer Biology and Management – An Introduction*, John Wiley and Sons, New York.

Yunis, J.J., 1983, The chromosome basis of human neoplasia, *Science,* **221**:227-236.

Zenser, T.V. and Coe, R.M., 1990, *Cancer and Aging – Progress in Research and Treatment*, Springer Verlag, New York.

Index

Aberrant differentiation, 50, 130
Achlorhydria, 55
Acquired immunodeficiency syndrome (AIDS), 120-122
Actinomycin D, 167
Activation, 17
Adenine (A), 18, 201
Adenocarcinoma, 184
Aflotoxin, 47, 48, 77
Aging, 125-128
Aging rate, 126
Agrobacterium tumefaciens, 140
AIDS virus, 121, 122, 180
Alcohol, 179
Alfa fetoprotein (AFP), 161
Amino acids, 21, 25, 26
Animals, 108
Animal fat, 77, 129, 137
Antibody, 151, 169
Antigen, 169, 170
Anti-oncogenes, 195
Apoptosis, 191
Aryl hydrocarbon hydralases (AHH), 90
Asbestos, 88, 129
Atomic bombs, 96, 102
Atomic bomb holocaust, 96, 179
Autosomal dominant, 55, 57

Beef fat, 178
Benign melanomas, 145, 147
Benign tumours, 14, 65
Benz(a)pyrene, 88, 90
Betel nut quid, 74
Betel quid cancer, 71
Binary fission, 202
Biochemical markers, 159, 163, 187
Bladder cancer, 47
Blood, 160
Blood groups, 16
Bone cancer, 70, 99, 103
Bone marrow cell, 30
Boveri, Theodore, 130
Brain cancer, 97, 179
Breast cancer, 53, 54, 56, 97, 117, 118, 135, 160, 170, 179

Burkitt's lymphoma, 64, 109, 133, 167

Caesium 137, 98, 99
Caffeine, 81
Cancer cells, 2, 3, 4, 12, 13, 30, 33, 35, 41, 45, 130, 154
Cancer detection, 3, 5, 6, 187, 209
Cancer genes, 203
Cancer of mouth, 48
Cancer predisposition, 183
Cancer prevention, 181
Cancer probands, 184
Cancer therapy, 160
Carcinoembryonic antigen (CEA), 160
Carcinogenesis, 115, 131, 134, 135, 208
Carcinogenic factors, 68, 69, 77, 80, 82, 92, 107, 174
Carcinogenic risk, 181
Carcinogens, 67, 88, 93, 107, 123, 129, 133, 156
Carcinoma, 14, 153
Cat, 112
Cell culture, 91
Cell cycle, 28, 37, 194
Cell death, 36, 43, 191
Cell differentiation, 6, 25, 26, 39, 40, 45, 101
Cell division, 12, 28, 31, 33, 194, 206
Cell fusion, 189
Cell growth, 39, 207
Cell replacement, 42, 191
Cell reproduction, 2, 25, 26, 101, 106, 130, 132, 203, 204
Cellular genes, 202
Cellular oncogenes, 101, 109, 111, 112, 115, 131
Cellular proto-oncogenes, 204, 208
Centromere, 33
Charcoal broiling, 81
Chemical carcinogenesis, 92-94
Chemotherapy, 167, 168
Chicken, 112
Chimney sweeps and scrotal cancer, 69, 89
Chloroplast, 10
Chromatids, 33
Chromatin network, 12
Chromosomes, 6, 10, 12, 16, 20, 26, 31, 57, 131, 189
  rearrangement of, 26
Chromosome number, 10
Chromosome abnormalities, 15, 61, 64, 65, 101, 103, 130
Chronic myelogenous leukaemia (CML), 63, 64
Cigar smoking, 76
Cigarette smoking, 4, 74, 76, 93
Clonal origin, 42, 128
Cloning, 202
Colon cancer, 55, 56, 57, 76, 78, 129, 135, 160, 184
Complementarity, 18
Complementary chains, 20
Contact inhibition, 155
Control of cancer, 1, 164, 165
Cri du chat syndrome, 61
Crown gall tumour, 140
Customs, 67, 71
Cyclin D1, 194
Cytokines, 192

Cytosine (C), 18, 201

DDT, 84
Defective genes, 4, 6, 15, 57
Deletion, 148, 158
Deoxyribonucleic acid (DNA), 12, 17, 18, 21, 26, 59, 92, 94, 106, 114, 122, 127, 131, 133, 201
Determination, 60
Detergents, 82
Development, 134, 135, 204
Developmental genetic programme, 126
Developmental phase, 134, 137, 140
Diet, 4, 76, 81, 129, 174, 177
Dietary factors, 55
Dietary fat, 54, 80, 178
Diethylstilbestrol (DES), 85, 171
Differentiation, 60, 132, 203, 204, 207
Dinosaurs, 1
DNA fingerprinting, 5
DNA replication, 28
DNA sequencing, 197
DNA synthesis, 28, 134
DNA template, 25
DNA virus, 108
Dominant gene, 58, 184
Dominantly inherited colon cancer, 186
Down's syndrome, 61
Drugs, 174, 179

Early detection, 158, 160
Egg nucleus, 39
Electrophiles, 89
Electron microscope, 8, 106
Embryo, 60
Endogenous mutagens, 127
Endoplasmic reticulum, 8, 13
Environmental carcinogens, 4, 15
Environmental factors, 47, 48, 54, 126, 129, 153, 174, 180, 194
Environmental pollutants, 67
Enzymes, 17
Epidemiological studies, 67, 174, 178, 180, 210
Epigenetic changes, 94, 130, 132, 135, 153, 204
Epstein-Barr virus, 109
Error-prone cells, 126
Estrogen, 85
Excision-repair genes, 59
Expression (*ee*) genes, 143

Feline leukaemia virus (FeLV), 120, 151
Fertilization, 39
Fibroblast, 155
'Fire drill,' 1, 169
Fish, 114, 178
Food additives, 80, 83, 210
Four periods, (G1, G2, S, and D), 28, 29, 35
Fragile sites, 62
Free radicals, 127

Gamma rays, 95, 97
Gardner's syndrome, 56
Gene-environment interaction, 17
Gene expression, 25
Gene mutation, 101, 102, 103, 133, 134,
Gene therapy, 197
Gene transfer, 199

Genetic aberrations, 5
Genetic change, 2, 4, 15, 127, 135, 153, 204
Genetic code, 18, 21, 23, 24, 26
Genetic components, 4
Genetic constellation, 141
Genetic constitution, 192
Genetic control, 126
Genetic counselling, 184, 186
Genetic defect, 5, 50
Genetic dictionary, 201
Genetic disease, 4, 5, 50, 130, 200
Genetic engineering, 141, 199, 200, 205
Genetic factors, 47, 50
Genetic information, 12
Genetic predisposition, 53
Genetic programme, 41, 191
Genetic tumours, 141
Genome structure, 197
Germ cells, 58
Glycoproteins, 161
Growth centres, 40
Guanine (G), 18, 201
Guinea pigs, 108, 112

Habits, 67, 71
Haemoglobin, 10, 17, 42
Half-life, 99
Hamster, 108, 112
HeLa cell line 154
Hepatitis B virus, 111
Hepatoma, 36
Hereditary cancers, 6, 183
Hereditary traits, 51, 53, 58
Heritable change, 26
Herpes virus, 16, 133, 180
Hiroshima, 96, 97, 102
Hodgkin's disease, 166
Hormones, 54, 140, 162
Hormone therapy, 170
Host range (of viruses), 108
Human cells, 91, 154, 156
Human chromosome(s), 8, 9, 11, 13, 14, 17, 21, 22, 54, 57, 61, 63, 64, 65
Human embryo, 34, 40
Human genome, 6, 16, 208
Human immunodeficiency virus (HIV), 120, 121, 122, 180
Human papilloma virus, 111
Human system, 153
Huntington's chorea, 5, 6
Hybridoma, 189
Hyperthermia, 1, 169

Iatrogenic weaponry, 13
Immortality, 191, 192, 193
Immune surveillance mechanism, 111, 208
Immune system, 15
Immunoadjuvants, 170
Immunological control, 169
Impairment, 25, 94
Incipient cancer genes, 202
Infrastructure, 205
Inherited diseases, 6
Inherited susceptibility, 117
Initiation, 92, 93, 134, 135, 204
Initiation phase, 134, 137, 140
Initiator (*I*), 143
Interferons, 171, 172
Interleukins, 172, 192
Invasive behaviour, 2, 5, 13, 14, 135
Inversion, 101

Iodine, 99
Ionizing radiation, 96, 102, 179
Irreversible cancer process, 133, 134, 135

Jumping genes, 190

Kanghri-burn cancer, 71
Kidney cancer, 170
Killer cells, 169

Latent period, 3, 75, 128, 158
Leukaemia, 2, 15, 30, 36, 43, 45, 64, 96, 97, 99, 102, 115, 118, 119, 133, 151, 164, 167, 179
Leukaemia viruses, 119, 120, 150
Life span, 36, 127, 191
Lifestyle, 181
Liver cancer, 47, 48, 50, 70, 76, 77, 99
Lung cancer, 4, 48, 74, 75, 76, 90, 93, 97, 129, 135, 164, 176
Lymphocytes, 151
Lymphoma, 15, 167

Malarial parasite, 3
Malignant adenocarcinoma, 55
Malignant melanoma, 145, 147
Malignant tumours, 14, 57, 64, 131
Mammary cancer, 149
Mammary tumour, 115, 117
Mammography, 100, 179
Maturation, 43
Meat consumption and cancer, 78, 79
Medicinal agents, 180
Melanin, 17, 44
Melanoblast, 44
Melanocyte, 44
Meningioma, 65
Mental retardation, 61
Messenger ribonucleic acid (mRNA), 21, 25, 135
Metastasis, 6, 13, 60, 135, 159
Mice, 108, 112, 119
Microbes, 2, 5
Microsomes, 89
Microwave radiation, 100
Milk (as a means of transmission), 116, 117, 118, 150
Mitochondria, 8, 133
Moderation, 180, 210
Molecular biology, 6
Molecular markers, 187
Monkey, 108
Mouse, 151, 152
Mouse cells, 156
Mouse mammary tumour virus (MMTV), 116, 150
Multicellular organisms, 1, 7, 42, 139, 201, 204
Multistep process, 134
Murine leukaemia virus (MLV), 150
Mutagens, 92
Mutation, 25, 26, 50, 58, 59, 94, 101, 109, 112, 115, 126, 132, 167, 202, 203
Myeloid leukaemia, 103

Nagasaki, 96, 97, 102
Natural killer cells, 111
Nerve cells, 41
Neutrons, 97, 102
Nitrites, 55, 80, 177, 178

Nitrosoamines, 80, 81, 178
Non-ionizing radiation, 96
Non-oncogenic viruses, 105, 106, 107
Normal cells, 6, 12, 13, 30, 34, 130, 154
Nuclear accidents and cancer, 98, 99
Nuclear fission, 98
Nucleolus, 10
Nucleophiles, 89
Nucleotides, 18
Nucleus, 7, 10
Nuclear power plants, 98

Occupational cancers, 69
Oncogene, 58, 112, 138, 188, 192, 193, 195, 200, 205
Oncogenic viruses, 105, 106, 107, 108, 122, 123
Oncogenic retroviruses, 113
Organelles, 8, 10
Origin of cancer, 129
Ovarian cancer, 193
Oxidants, 127

P^{53}, 195, 196
Pernicious anaemia, 55
Pesticides, 73, 82, 84, 90
Pigment cells, 144, 145
Philadelphia chromosome, 62, 63, 64
Plasma membrane, 7
Platyfish, 144, 145, 147, 148
Polarity, 20
Pollutants, 68, 210
Polycyclic hydrocarbons, 69
Polymerase chain reaction (PCR), 6
Polyoma virus, 108
Polyposis of the colon, 55
Polyps, 56, 184
Position effect, 133
Preservatives, 74
Preventable cancers, 60, 69, 174, 176
Prevention of cancer, 106, 174, 184, 208, 209
Programmed cell death, 191, 192
Promiscuity, 179, 180
Prostate acid phosphatase (PAP), 161
Prostate-specific antigen (PSA), 161
Protective genes, 50
Proteins, 5, 17, 162
Protein synthesis, 21, 126
Proto-oncogenes, 63, 64, 66, 115, 137, 144
Purines, 18
Pyrimidines, 18

Radioactive fallout, 98
Radioactivity, 99
Radiation, 73, 95, 100, 101, 129, 132, 156, 165, 166, 174
Radiation therapy, 167
Radium, 99
Radon, 95
Random amplified polymorphic DNA (RAPD), 198
Rat, 108, 112, 119
Recombinant DNA technology, 141, 172, 199

Red blood cells, 41, 127
Regulatory genes (R-genes), 25, 50, 94, 115, 123, 130, 131, 133, 134, 137, 138, 147, 188, 189, 195, 203, 205
Repeated DNA, 193, 203
Replication, 202
Replicator, 193, 203
Resting nucleus, 12
Restriction enzymes, 198
Restriction fragment length polymorphism (RFLP), 6, 198
Retinoblastoma, 15, 57, 58, 135, 166
  non-hereditary, 57, 58
Retroviruses, 112, 114, 115, 117, 133, 150, 199
Reverse transcriptase, 112, 120, 133
Reversible cancer, 132
Rhabdomyosarcoma, 168
Rhesus factor, 16
Ribosomes, 8, 10
Ribonucleic acid (RNA), 21, 106, 114, 201
RNA tumour viruses, 112, 123
Rous sarcoma virus (RSV), 114

Salmonella, 92
Sarcoma, 15, 114
Screening, 91, 187, 209
Scrotal cancer, 69, 89
Selective matings, 148
Self-destruction, 14
Senescence, 127
Sex cells, 60
Sex chromosomes, 10, 39, 61
Sickle cell anaemia, 5
Skin cancer, 5, 45, 47, 48, 59, 69, 72, 93, 99, 103, 164, 177
Smoking and cancer, 90, 98, 99
Solid tumours, 15
Somatic cells, 58
Somatic mutations, 65, 131
Spindle apparatus, 33
Spot-specific loci, 145
Staphylococcus, 3
Stem cells, 42, 45, 152
Sterilization, 185
Stomach cancer, 47, 54, 56, 76, 81, 129, 135, 177, 178
Stresses, 141
Substitution, 26
Sunlight, 5, 48, 99, 177
Suppression, 17
Suppressor genes (*see also* tumour suppressor genes), 60, 66, 101, 103, 130, 131, 138, 193, 195, 200, 204, 208
Surgery, 165, 167
Susceptibility genes, 54
Swordtail (fish), 144, 145, 147, 148

Telomerase, 192, 193
Telomeres, 193
Teratocarcinoma, 151, 152
Therapeutic drugs, 82
Thorium, 99
Thorotrast, 99
Three-dimensional growth, 202, 203, 204
Thymine (*T*), 18, 201
Thyroid cancer, 97, 179

Tissue-specific genes, 131, 133
Tissue-specific regulatory genes, 204
Tobacco, 74, 141, 174
Tobacco smoke, 90, 129
Tobacco smoking, 75, 76, 176
Totipotent, 152
Transfer RNA (tRNA), 25
Transformation, 3, 4, 6, 89, 115, 123, 130. 140, 153, 154, 155, 156, 171
Transforming genes (*Tr*), 111, 131
Translocation, 63, 64, 101
Transposable elements, 190
Treatment, 1, 165
Tumour, 1, 91, 93, 108, 130, 135, 139, 144, 151, 156, 159, 166, 169, 171
Tumour (T) antigen, 123, 170
Tumour gene (*Tu*), 131
Tumourigenesis, 137
Tumour-prone tissues, 60
Tumour suppressor genes, 58, 194, 196
Twins and CML, 62

Ultraviolet rays (radiation), 4, 5, 26, 44, 48, 50, 96, 99, 103, 129
Unicellular forms, 202
Unrestrained cell reproduction, 2
Uracil (U), 21
Uranium, 98
Urine, 162
Urinary bladder cancer, 70

Vaccine (for AIDS), 122
Viral oncogenesis, 112, 132, 133
Viruses, 4, 54, 129, 156, 202

Wilm's tumour, 167, 168
White blood cells (leucocytes), 15, 45, 63, 119

Xeroderma pigmentosum, 4, 15, 59, 60, 135
X-irradiation, 141
X-rays, 4, 26, 50, 84, 85, 97, 100, 102, 148

Zygote, 40, 60